D1547886

THUS
WE ARE MEN

THUS
WE ARE MEN

BY
SIR WALTER LANGDON-BROWN

Essay Index Reprint Series

 BOOKS FOR LIBRARIES PRESS
FREEPORT, NEW YORK

First Published 1938
Reprinted 1969

STANDARD BOOK NUMBER:
8369-1148-2

LIBRARY OF CONGRESS CATALOG CARD NUMBER:
79-86768

PRINTED IN THE UNITED STATES OF AMERICA

To My Collaborator :

MY WIFE

CONTENTS

vii

PREFACE

This book largely consists of addresses delivered before different audiences, but revision, addition, and excision have been freely practised where it seemed advisable. I am indebted to the Editors of the following journals :— *The St. Bartholomew's Hospital Journal, The Journal of Mental Science, The British Medical Journal, The Lancet, The Listener* and the *West London Medico-Chirurgical Journal,* for kindly permitting me to reprint contributions to their columns. I trust I have also made adequate acknowledgment in the text of my indebtedness to the authors from whom I have so freely quoted, and whose thoughts I have found so stimulating.

THUS
WE ARE MEN

INTRODUCTION

" Thus we are men and we know not how " ; so wrote Sir Thomas Browne three centuries ago. Nor do we really know to-day, though there has never been a time when it was possible to obtain so wide a view of man's position in the universe. We can even put a limit to space, though we can form no conception of what lies outside it. Space itself is so vast that we can only dimly appreciate it in terms of the years that light must take to traverse it. Turning from this enormous vista to regard the minutest atom, we find within a whirl of electrons which has revolutionized our ideas of matter and energy. Turning again from space to time, whereas the mental vision of our grandfathers was limited to a mere six thousand years, we can in imagination watch the slow condensation of a nebula to make a world, the formation of its land and water, and the gradual evolution of life upon it through countless æons until man appears. We can watch his struggles, his falls and advances, his potentialities for good and evil. Finally through his reactions to the physical and mental sufferings induced by the War and its sequels we have arrived at a much clearer conception of what is man.

Everyone knows that we are living on a thin crust of solid earth lying over lava and a fiery furnace, but the man who has felt the earth rock under his feet or has looked into the crater of a volcano realizes that fact with a vividness to which no philosophical recognition can attain. And those of us who have seen civilization rock and its landmarks disappear, can realize in a way that our parents could not that under the thin crust of civilization ages of savage passion still boil and burn.

Attaining a view-point often entails considerable discomfort, not to say risk ; we are living in an uncomfortable, perhaps dangerous, age and must get what compensation we can by interesting ourselves in the extensive view before us, in which there may be faintly discernible " the shape of things to come ".

I have described in this book some of the view-points which have attracted and interested me in the course of my professional career and have attempted to present them in a form which might be described as a theme with variations. The main theme may be briefly defined thus. As we are animals we conform to biological laws. Our further evolution physically is improbable and mentally unlikely. Therefore only a psychological evolution remains. This necessitates co-operation, not merely instinctive as with the bees and ants, but intelligent and voluntary. Now we, like all animals, carry with us vestigial traces of our past ancestry, not least in our mental processes. To develop psychologically we must understand ourselves, and it should help us to do so if we can find ways to investigate those hidden depths in our minds from which we draw our impulses. One might draw a parallel between the processes of thought and of respiration. In ordinary breathing tidal air goes in and out. With an effort we can draw in complemental air and breathe out supplemental air, but there is always residual air remaining in the lungs. But this residual air by diffusion influences the composition of the others. The conscious level may be compared with tidal air, the sub-conscious with the complemental and supplemental air, while the unconscious resembles the residual air alike in being beyond the control of the will and in influencing, nevertheless, the higher levels.

Just as the physiologist has his methods of analysing the residual air in the lungs, so the psychologist has his ways of analysing the content of the unconscious mind. He can gather evidence from the growing mind of a child, for just as the embryo rehearses our earlier physical states, modified by a different environment, so in childhood the mind repeats earlier mental states modified by helplessness and dependence. He can also obtain medical evidence. The more recently a characteristic has been acquired, the more easily is it disturbed by physical disease or mental distress. In either case the sufferer tends to revert to a more primitive mode of thought. The truth underlying the old saying *in vino veritas* is that with the removal of self control the primitive man reappears, modified by intoxication.

There is yet another means of approach—the study of works of creative imagination. As Marc Semenoff expresses it: " Literature, music, sculpture, painting, and architecture can help man to psycho-analyse himself."

The theme itself is by no means new, but I hope that the variations I have composed may be of interest even though my own sympathies and antipathies must unavoidably strike some recurring notes. In the first place I have tried to relate man to his social environment. There is inevitably some conflict not only between the interest of the individual and that of the herd but, as we know full well, between the interests of different herds. For here arises opposition between two powerful tendencies ; on the one hand the evolutionary demand for enlargement of the unit, on the other the species-making impulse which makes for segregation. It is only to be expected that a community would evolve more slowly than the individuals of which it is composed ; indeed, international troubles largely arise from the fact that different communities do not reach the same evolutionary level at the same time. There is also the regressive influence of the past in delaying progress ; unfavourable genes have their effect as well as the favourable ones. I have maintained that evolution always offers both a higher and a lower road, but its inexorable sentence is " modify or disappear " when the organism is confronted by a changing environment.

Since reason is a more recent acquisition than emotion, it is not surprising that distresses whether of the individual or of the community tend to produce a revolt against reason. This is discussed under the title " We have reason to think ". After all Reason was man's charioteer in the vision of Socrates, and so should remain. Reason also permits imitative play as a training ; make-believe is a preparation for reality, if only it is recognized as such. Thus intelligence comes to replace the automatic responses of instinct ; if less certain, it is more adaptable to new situations and the path is thereby opened to higher developments. It is true that reason cannot explain everything, but that is no excuse for taking nonsense as a guide. That the deeper levels of the mind have an aptitude for distorting ideas into nonsense our dreams sufficiently prove. This leads me to a discussion of the aims of medicine and of certain impediments to its progress under the title of " The Return of Æsculapius ". For I believe the trend of twentieth century medicine is towards a revival of the best features of Greek ideals.

About a dozen years ago some bronze statues were dredged up off the coast of Greece. They had lain at the bottom of the sea ever since the wreck of the ship that was carrying them to Rome in the days of Hadrian. I watched one of them being carefully cleaned and dried in the Museum at Athens. It was an exquisitely beautiful figure of a boy, perfect in every respect except for the palm of his left hand. His right arm was uplifted and he appeared to be gazing with wonder and delight at something which has now vanished, but once rested on that left hand. It has been suggested that this was a lyre which the boy had struck and that he stood there enchanted by the music he had created. Or it may well have been that he was gazing intently on some wonder of the deep which he had found. For me it was a symbol of the recurrent wonder and delight that different generations have experienced on discovering again the treasures of the Greek mind which more than once have sunk beneath a sea of indifference and neglect.

Pathology is essentially a study of the reactions which the body makes when faced by an abnormal situation ;

4

psychopathology is the same process applied to the reactions of the mind, though the more we consider man as a psychosomatic unity the better. The compensations which are made for such situations are a guide to the working of the human mind, and help not only the medical man to understand the mechanisms of neurosis, but also the individual to make the appropriate adaptations once the position is made clear to him. The neurotic will nevertheless have to work out his own salvation. Others may be needed to find the path, but he will have to tread it himself, however steep it may be. This he is often unwilling to do. He may, indeed, accept the logic of his psychotherapist's conclusions, but maintain that he would prefer the shelter which his neurosis affords rather than face the world without it. The origins and manifestations of some typical neuroses are discussed under the titles of "Just Nerves", "New Pains for Old", and "The Style of Life". It may be asked how can such studies help us to adjust ourselves to life? To this Professor Tansley supplies the answer. "It has become almost a commonplace that man is not primarily a rational being, though it is by the use of reason alone that he can attain in any degree to the mastery of his destiny. He still relies on reason only where its usefulness is forcibly and immediately brought home to him. For the most part he is a passionate and credulous creature, the slave of his instincts and of the suggestions arising from his instincts, or from the most dubious external sources which may simulate authority. It is remarkable, when these plain facts are considered, how widespread in much of the writing supposed to instruct and direct us is the tacit assumption that man *is* primarily a rational creature, that he may contentedly neglect the study of his origins, of the real nature of his instincts and of the devious paths they pursue, of the hidden motives by which he is generally driven, and that he may safely face the world and the complicated problems of modern life relying upon the childish belief that his mind is simple, rational, and straightforward."

The next section of this book is devoted mainly to an attempt at interpreting the writings of certain authors as a revelation of the workings of the unconscious mind. Lord Balfour once said that what he most dreaded was being " explained ", and it may well be that the authors in question would not have agreed with my explanations of their art. Nor are they here to defend themselves. Still I do not take such an extreme position as Lenormand, when he says : " I do not believe that one can decide the relations between the artist and his art by identifying the two but rather by setting them in opposition to one another. . . . Sometimes the piece of art rises up against the artist like a child rebelling against his father. Often the artist contemplates his work with the astonished gaze which an honest man might cast upon a son who has turned out a criminal, pondering on the defects he has transmitted without being tainted himself. . . . The work of art is only a discharge of the unconscious obsessions of the artist. . . . It is unlikely that he would ever commit the deeds of his characters . . . The writer exorcises his demons in describing them."

There is an element of truth in this, but it is not the whole truth. It does, however, explain the violent contrast often found between the artist and the art he creates. But I would claim for the greatest art that it embodies so much of the universal mind, that the beholder finds in it the reflection of something in his own mind. Of art as of everything in life it is true that what we find in it depends largely on what we bring to it.

I have illustrated this part of my theme by several references to seventeenth century literature, not only because it has always interested me to try and discover why men thought what they did when they did, but also because the post-Victorian age seems to be confronted with rather similar problems to those of the post-Elizabethan age. In this section I have also brought to my support the powerful aid of Dr. Robert Bridges, whose *Testament of Beauty* states poetically and far more

6

aptly than I can many of the ideas I have tried to express. He may well be claimed as the Poet of Evolution.

The third section is more miscellaneous. I do not anticipate that many will agree with the views expressed in " Some Gods and their Makers ", since it is an attempt to trace the evolution of the religious impulse. Those who regard religion as revealed will frankly disapprove; those who regard it as mere superstition will disagree with my conclusions ; to both theological and classical scholars, should any such read this, it must appear rather an amateur effort. My defence must be that I wrote it chiefly to clarify my impressions for myself, and so I hope that some like-minded may find it of interest and even helpful. I have also applied the evolutionary idea to Italian Art, in order to illustrate the fact that the processes of growth and decay are as inevitable for the creations of the human mind as for man himself. This is true even though, as I point out, biology teaches us that death is not inherent in life itself, but is evolved by life for the good of the species.

" Man is a noble animal, splendid in ashes and pompous in the grave, solemnizing nativities and deaths with equal lustre." " Thus we are men and we know not how : there is something in us that can be without us, and will be after us ; though it is strange that it hath no history what it was before us."

I

THE BIOLOGY OF SOCIAL LIFE

THE BIOLOGY OF SOCIAL LIFE[1]

I appreciate very deeply the honour of being invited to deliver this, the seventeenth, Maudsley Memorial Lecture. I also feel the responsibility of adequately fulfilling a task, so well carried out by my predecessors and so brilliantly initiated by Sir James Crichton-Browne. I never had the privilege of knowing Henry Maudsley, but Sir James's description of his fellow Yorkshireman as having " a dash of Wuthering Heights about him " illuminated him for me as by a flash of lightning. It has been said that his last book, *Organic to Human,* embodies his philosophy which may be summed up in the principle of unity of the human organism and its continuity with the rest of Nature's processes. His *Pathology of Mind* also bears abundant testimony to his deep and life-long interest in the subject on which with some temerity I am venturing to address you. Whether I should have been rash enough to do so in his presence is another matter. I recall the fate of " a certain clergyman " whom Dr. Samuel Johnson blasted into silence by a single thunderbolt, and I fear that Dr. Henry Maudsley's keen and logical mind would descry some loose joints in my argument. So I crave your indulgence.

I have taken as my title " The Biology of Social Life ". It is obvious that man, being a social animal, will be subject to the biological laws which govern life in general and gregarious animals in particular. Yet how generally that simple fact is forgotten, although Wilfred Trotter has dealt, in his usual masterly style, with the

[1] The seventeenth Maudsley lecture delivered before the Royal Medico-Psychological Association, 25th November, 1936.

11

instincts of the herd, and Morley Roberts with admirable skill has traced many biological and sociological parallels. I must acknowledge my indebtedness to them both by saying how stimulating their point of view has been to me.

Looking at the film made by the late Dr. Canti of the growth of bone under a microscope, one is struck by the ceaseless activity of the cells, busily engaged in building round the girders which are shooting out in all directions. Watching their apparently purposeful behaviour, it seems that when we say " my body ", we are speaking rather as a king does when he says " my country " or " my subjects ". Indeed, we know even less of the behaviour of our constituent cells than he does of the lives and deaths, the hopes and fears, the hates and loves of those over whom he rules.

It is a biological axiom that life started as a single cell, and still continues to do so. The most striking thing about a living cell is its incessant urge to assert itself as strongly as its environment will permit. This is the real struggle for existence. It is an extraordinarily interesting fact that if embryonic kidney cells, for instance, are grown by themselves in a suitable medium they appear, according to some observers, to become positively malignant. Put some embryonic connective tissue into that medium and the kidney cells promptly conform to type. They have to learn to adapt themselves to the needs of their neighbour. Cancer is a process of cell anarchy, the malignant cell brutally riding rough-shod over the others. Just so a man sufficiently released from the control of his environment becomes malignant, like many autocrats. As Lord Baldwin said : " None of us is wise enough or good enough to be a dictator."

Maudsley wrote : " It is not easy for the individual to realize how much he owes to the restraints and supports of the social fabric in which he is an element, and which, like the atmosphere, always and insensibly surrounds him. There could not be a greater danger to the balance of any mind than to be exempt from the bonds and pressure of the surrounding social system." We see that contention of his illustrated in the United States to-day where, although one is particularly conscious of the pressure of herd opinion, there are outbreaks of gangster-dom, chiefly among imported aliens who have been set free from their own environment, but have not assimilated themselves with the new, remaining Ishmaelites, within it. It is one of the drawbacks of these vast new suburbs, mere dormitories, which radiate out like huge tentacles from London, destroying the countryside as they grow, that they offer so few opportunities for communal life and a social background.

The whole story of many-celled organisms is one of mutual adjustments between the different tissues, each trying to do its best for itself within the limits of those adjustments. The first stage in evolution was a number of single cells herding together for mutual support but each doing the same work. The next stage was one when groups of cells did different work. In evolution there are two parallel processes—increasing division of labour and increasing co-ordination between the different parts. The latter was achieved under the control of the central nervous system. A strong central government is needed to help to keep order, and no high degree of differentiation is possible in the animal body without the control of a centralized nervous system which has gradually acquired an increasing predominance. It is not too fanciful to compare the origin of the nervous system to a group of settlers on the coast who gradually invade the interior, first singly and then in an organized army, as in the nervous system of vertebrates, which arises as a tube on the surface of the body. Once established the invader assumes control over the indigenous inhabitants, fortifying itself as it goes, and maintaining its protectorate by a system of rapid communication throughout the invaded areas. The biological and sociological parallel is remarkably complete.

Just as the cells struggle to achieve the best they can within their environment, so the individual they form struggles either to do so, or to change its surroundings. The mud-fish gasping for breath on the mud-flats and struggling to reach the land was, no doubt, actuated by the need to escape from the competition of life in the sea towards the abundant food supply on the land. From that successful struggle all the land vertebrates and ultimately man himself arose. The power motive is therefore inherent in every cell in our body and is inherited from our remotest ancestors.

Now, in the evolution of the invertebrates a terrible difficulty arose—they are so constructed that their nervous systems cannot develop further without choking them. In the invertebrates with the most developed brains the mouth is so closely encircled by the nervous system that they have, perforce, to confine their feeding to blood-sucking. Hence the dilemma between having sufficient intelligence to secure food, and adequate capacity to consume it. Two methods of escape from the dilemma were found—one the development of the gregarious habit ; the other the new pattern of nervous system which characterizes the vertebrate. The former method, in which each individual is absorbed into the community and is helpless apart from it, marks an advance which was fraught with great possibilities. For bees and ants this was comparatively easy, because of the very smallness of the brain of the individual and the limited number of reactions of which it is capable. Moreover, the social habit in insects has imposed its demands, not only on the work but on the structure of the individuals composing the group. It has sterilized large numbers, rendering them neuter and thus enormously simplifying the problem. Conflict and competition are greatly increased in a community where each individual aims at seeing himself immortalized in his offspring. Still more is this the case when one such community comes up against another similar one. The evolution of the vertebrate gave ample opportunities for the brain to expand. As the higher centres developed, the automatic actions of the lower centres were held in check while more skilled voluntary movements became possible. And as the highest level developed it exercised control over both voluntary and automatic movements, restraining emotional expression but increasing skill through increased intelligence. Thus man, having laboriously acquired the power of speech, had to learn the still more subtle art of silence.

But long before man appeared another " fault " in evolution had occurred. The first was the dilemma between nutrition and intelligence among the invertebrates ; the second was in the development of the mesozoic reptiles, in which the central nervous system was too rudimentary to control so huge a frame. Lord Samuel made some amusing play not long ago with the idea of such animals having an elaborate system of protection such as so often went with scanty brain power and drew some political parallels consonant with his own views. The complete disappearance of these enormous animals (except perhaps from Loch Ness !) recalls how frequently the worship of the ideal of the colossal has heralded a downfall. There is something about them that inevitably suggests the 'prentice hand— just as there is about the first railway engine, the first motor car, or the first " tank ". Anyhow, mere bigness was then exploited to the full and found wanting. Now it is important to note that on both these occasions a way of escape was found in gregariousness—the substitution of co-operation between smaller individuals, firstly for increased complexity of brain, and secondly for mere increased size of body.

The course of successful evolution has been to increase, not the size of the cell or of the individual, but of the unit. The unicellular became the multicellular ; isolated individuals became a community. For the mammal this was a much longer, more painful and more dangerous path than for the insect, just because its brain was capable of so many different reactions. This applies in an altogether special degree to man.

The first law of the herd is " Thou shalt not ". Just

as the development of the higher nerve centres checks instinctive activities, so the development of communal life must restrict the freedom of the individual. Man has not found this easy. Philosophers may lament this, theologians may attribute it to original sin, but the biologist will remember that the cells of which he is composed did not find it easy to sink their individuality in that of the organism. A clever woman once said to me of her son : " He hasn't fused his ancestors yet." It was profoundly true.

Yet evolution continues to demand that we shall fuse our ancestors, that we shall enlarge the unit. The family becomes the tribe, the tribe the small nation. The heptarchy becomes the monarchy, the nation an empire. And all the time the individuals within the unit are clamouring for self-expression, the smaller unit within the empire for self-determination. Sir Arthur Keith has called attention to two opposing tendencies in life —one the general demand for enlargement of the unit —the other, the species-making impulse which attempts to segregate a particular type. The first in human life makes for internationalism, the second for nationalism.

The recent fierce fanatical outbreak of nationalism becomes comprehensible as a frightened response of the species-making segregating impulse against the resistless imperious demand of the ever-widening evolutionary process towards internationalism. More and more, nations become interdependent, the health and prosperity of one affecting the health and prosperity of all. Just as the revolt of the members against the belly became the defeat of all, so war has become a process in which all can lose but none gain. To win a war to-day is a greater disaster than it formerly was to lose one. Norman Angell pointed that out years ago ; war would have been impossible if man were a rational animal. But to claim that man is a rational animal is to express a wish rather than to state a fact. Man is not a rational animal, though he may be in process of becoming so. But though reason is not the parent of many of his actions, he seeks reason for their god-parent, by trying to find reasonable explanations for what his emotions drive him to do. He prefers to ignore the savage ancestry of his unconscious mind. The outlook for increasing internationalism which we hoped for after the War is being replaced by a mentality resembling that of the Dobu islanders in Melanesia, whose slogan is: "If your yams flourish, mine will rot." In many respects popular ideas and ideals are undergoing a perilous repression. Here may I draw an analogy from Freud's doctrine concerning such repressions ? If this species-making impulse is, as I think, repressing the evolutionary trend towards the expansion of the unit, one might expect that trend to take an abnormal course. The building up of vertical walls between nations is being countered by horizontal lines of cleavage, which threaten to divide Europe into Fascists and Communists. This, to my mind, represents the pathological form of internationalism resulting from repression of its normal expression.

Just as the nervous system must be developed to allow of sufficiently rapid co-operation between the various organs of the individual, so means of rapid communications are essential to co-ordination of the complex civilization of to-day. It has been truly said " civilization *is* communication ". One of the many factors in the downfall of the Roman Empire was the inadequacy of the methods of communication for the size it had attained. And so it suffered the fate of the mesozoic reptile. This difficulty does not obtain to-day. Means of communication could be excellent ; so the forces which would oppose evolution offer artificial barriers to free communication—passports, visas, and the like. And all the time the development of aviation is making frontiers as obsolete as the octroi and the toll-gate. Indeed, the great ease of communication by wireless is having some interesting effects. At first the leader could address personally all the members of a small tribe. The Greeks considered that the size of a city state was limited by the number of freemen who could assemble in a given place. Then as States increased in size various methods were evolved of appointing representatives of large groups to act for them. In democratic countries political power gradually passed into the hands of such representatives. But now the ruler can speak by wireless to a vast audience, which has facilitated a return to absolutism. We learned in the General Strike in 1926 what a powerful weapon wireless placed in the hands of the government, and dictators have not been slow to avail themselves of it.

In disease of the body the higher levels which develop last suffer first, for they have not had time to acquire such a firm hold on the instincts of the organism as the lower. In the same way the body politic evolves its higher levels later than the individuals composing it. A committee is always more ready to perpetrate an injustice than its individual members would be. The laws of a nation may be fixed, but its ideas of international law are varied to suit its convenience. A contract between individuals may be indefeasible ; a treaty between nations is not. The contract may be enforced by superior authority ; the observance of a treaty, up to the present, has depended on force of arms. Yet this is no more logical than the settlement of a private quarrel by a duel. That it should be wrong for the individual to kill but right for the State to do so can only represent a transitional state in evolution. But in national affairs the human mind is still obsessed by the fallacy of force, though it has realized that in private affairs right does not necessarily lie with the better shot.

If we cannot adapt ourselves to the demands of evolution the issue is not in doubt. This civilization will go as others have gone. Flinders Petrie, in his fascinating little book on *The Revolutions of Civilization*, maintains that we are now in the eighth cycle of civilization. Each previous one has waxed and waned and a dark age has intervened before the rise of the next. He regards as the real sign of progress throughout the ages the fact that the summers of the civilized periods are getting longer and the winters of the dark ages in between are getting shorter. He points out that the rise of each new civilization has originated "from a mixture of two different stocks. That effect of mixture cannot take place all at once. There are barriers of antipathy, barriers of creed, barriers of social standing, but every barrier of race fusion gives away in time when two races are in contact". History gives many illustrations of the truth of this. Romeo and Juliet will always be impelled to break down the barriers between Montagus and Capulets. The classic civilization of the Greeks arose from the blending of a Northern with a Mediterranean stock. The Normans, a blending of Norsemen with Latins, were building cathedrals which are our admiration to-day at a time when their Scandinavian forbears were still building little wooden churches. Normandy, England, and Sicily assumed new importance at their hands. With all the facts of the advantages of interbreeding at our disposal, how paltry and jejune is all this chatter about pure Nordic races which besets our ears to-day !

There are three stages in the evolution of human society ; to the first the name of " co-consciousness" has been applied or, as Aldrich calls it, " a collective uncon-scious morality inherent in the laws of life," so far as they can be appreciated. At this stage man is bound with a hypnotic completeness to every taboo. If he breaks a taboo he may even die, apparently from the sense of sin and isolation he experiences, as a bee dies when separated from the swarm. Rivers' studies of the Melanesians convinced him that they seemed to recognize instinctively, using that much-abused word in the strict sense, what the general feeling of the group was, and what definite line of action it should take. Such communities are stable precisely because they are not individualized. The avoidance of collisions between foot passengers in crowded pathways, thought reading, and social tact he regarded as vestiges among us to-day of that social common consciousness.

In the second stage individuals begin to emerge, and it is interesting to the medical profession to observe that

19

it is the witch doctor, the magician, who is the first to do so. As Gerald Heard says, probably the proto-individual realizes that he is different from the herd before it becomes apparent to them. So he adopts a rôle which is impressive to the onlooker and suggestive to himself. But he is soon conscious not only that he is alone, and that he can never go back, but that there is enmity between him and the tribe, which spares him because it fears him. He evolves into the priest-king and as Freud says, the elaborate taboos by which the lives of the priest-kings are made little better than a pestered imprisonment, are the outcome of a profound sub-conscious jealousy, based on a feeling of fundamental difference in quality between the group and this particular individual. Frazer inquires, why did it become customary in many parts of the world to put divine kings and other human gods to a violent death? It was because they feared that if they allowed him to die of sickness or of old age, his divine spirit might share in the weakness of its bodily tabernacle, or perhaps perish altogether, thereby entailing the most serious danger to the whole body of the tribe. Whereas by putting him to death while he was yet in full vigour of body and mind, they could transmit his still uncorrupted powers to his successors. This is the real origin of the divinity that doth hedge a king, who was at first a sacrificial object—the central object of fertility rites on which the survival of the tribe depended. But as the evolution of human society proceeds the individual learns to outwit the tribe, and to substitute others, or even an image or symbol for his own body, which was intended for sacrifice. Another man or an animal died in the king's stead. "The King is dead, long live the King." Such a change made for absolutism. The divine right went on without its distressing consequences.

This conception of kingship makes much more intelligible the ascription of divine powers and the final deification of the Cæsars for this was merely a reversion to an earlier mode of thinking. It also explains their frequent assassination, which must often have seemed a religious duty to the assassin. Even to-day in many parts of the world assassination of the ruler is too often regarded as a political argument, and lunatics, who are admittedly prone to revert to primitive methods of thought, find a particular fascination in it.

The king at this stage in his attempts to outwit the tribe realizes that what they want is physical plenty, and so he leads them out to conquest. A study of epic literature reveals that they are the record of a short, violent, vivid period in the advance of human culture, an invariable stage, the heroic age. There is a transition from the cult of the totem animal to the heroic cult. " The glorious heroes are for the most part kings, but not in the old sense, bound to the soil, responsible for its fertility. Homage paid them is devotion for personal character. . . . Another noticeable point is that in heroic poems scarcely anyone is safely and quietly at home." An heroic age is an almost invariable character-istic of the movements of people and comes to an end with their resettlement. We can therefore see how inevitable it is, even in modern times, that when a king claims divine right and leads his people out to battle unsuccessfully he should lose his crown, and often his head with it.

" The raiding stage over, the resettled peoples will, to some extent, return to magic, as they will have gone back to crop-raising, and will once again be obsessed with fertility ; the generalship will break up ; a separation arises between the priestly and the kingly aspects. On the religious side, priesthood will re-establish itself, but as a profession. This priesthood will not have to pay its old price, neither will it be paid the old reverence" (Gerald Heard). The struggles between the kingly and priestly aspects of rulers are typified in the Middle Ages by the recurring conflicts between Emperor and Pope. They were seen in Egypt in the conflict between the " modernist " Aknaton and the priests of the temples. If the priest wins, he puts a boyish usurper on the throne whom he can control. Such was Tut-ankh-Amen, who succeeded Aknaton. Seen from this angle what a fascinating story the history of the Old Testament becomes. Moses, followed by the victorious raiding general, Joshua ; the struggles between Samuel and Saul ; the successful claim of the priest to decide certain things against the king, as when Samuel hewed Agag in pieces before the Lord, but against the wish of Saul ; Saul, bewildered and outwitted by superior intelligence, reverts to fertility rites and consults the witch of Endor, and finally Samuel places the boyish usurper on the throne—David.

Originally only the king was regarded as having a future life, and therefore as the only one to possess a soul. But as individualism grew and spread, there was a similar demand from many humbler beings for immortality after death. Hence arose the mystery religions such as those of Osiris in Egypt, Orpheus in Greece, and Mithras in Persia, each of which purported to teach man how to attain to a future life. The spread of the Roman Empire imported these ideas into Rome itself where, especially in the second century, they contested fiercely for supremacy with Christianity. And no impartial observer can deny that Christianity in winning absorbed some of the tenets of its rivals. St. Paul sometimes used the exact phraseology of Osiris and the Eleusinian mysteries, and hymnology, particularly Cowper's, is steeped in Mithraism. At the co-conscious stage the individual is satisfied with the continuance of the tribe, and fertility rites satisfy his religious aspirations. But at the stage of individualism he demands personal immortality. Fertility rites are regarded with grave disfavour and even disgust, and man's religious aspirations are fixed upon the next world. " In Israel Josiah ends the fertility-religion with that sudden passionate revulsion against procreative rites which always attends such a termination, and which must show an abrupt amnesia of its own past."

And so individualism spreads and grows. In this second stage, as Aldrich says: " The group represses egotistic tendencies by forcibly imposing a conventional morality." But as more and more individuals become self-conscious the state becomes more unstable. It has been said that civilizations do not really decay, but burst from the tension produced by the rapid expansion of individualities within its borders. This is the present and urgent problem of civilization—to give scope for individual development, and yet for the individual to fit into his place as a part of a much larger whole. It is Aldrich's third stage—not yet reached by any society but recognized by an increasing number of persons—a stage in which the members of the group consciously co-operate for the common good, and not merely instinctively as in the social insects.

Heard emphasizes the point that whereas the first stage is accompanied by a fertility religion, while the second or individualistic stage is characterized by a religion in which personal salvation and personal immortality are the keynotes, neither of these is adequate for the third stage of conscious co-operation. Harold Nicolson considers that a struggle for world power creates conditions under which a new religion arises. And to-day far removed as we are from a new world state, a new religion of the state as an object of worship is rapidly growing up. In Germany the old gods of Valhalla are being decorated with the armour of knighthood, just as during the War the wooden image of Hindenburg was erected as a totem figure into which nails were symbolically driven. The anti-religious attitude of Russia is upheld with a fanatical and intensely religious fervour, and all over Europe, Fascism and Communism are fiercely competing religions.

Yet amid all change the human mind always desires to crystallize what should remain a living force, heedless of biology, which teaches that this is impossible. A living thing must always be changing—to crystallize is to kill the spirit and merely to preserve the letter. The human mind works with symbols, and as time goes on it is apt to take the symbol for the substance, instead of regarding it as an attempt, suited to the mentality of the age, to give expression to ideas otherwise intangible. Nowhere is this more clearly seen than in a comparative study of religions. With the flux of time the old symbolic representation becomes unacceptable and often frankly repulsive to many individuals in subsequent generations. Yet to many they represent the faith delivered once and for all, which it is sacrilege to question. Leonard Woolf puts it forcibly when he says: " The strangest and most important fact about communal psychology is that its content is largely the ideas, beliefs, and aims of the dead ... the law of the mortmain or the dead hand. . . . There can be no understanding of history, of politics, or of the effects of communal psychology which does not take into consideration the tremendous effect of this psychological dead hand, the dead mind. . . . At every particular moment it is the dead rather than the living who are making history, for politically individuals think dead men's thoughts and pursue dead men's ideals ... mere ghosts of beliefs, ideals from which time has sapped all substance and meaning. . . . A dogma is simply a belief which the living receive as a command from the dead."

But I would suggest that the real reason why this influence which the dead past continues to exert over the living man is so powerful, is that he carries within himself, still living, the genes of his dead ancestors. For, as Samuel Butler said in *Life and Habit* : " His past selves are living in him at this moment with the accumulated life of centuries. ' Do this, this, this, which we too have done and found profit in it,' cry the souls of his forefathers within him. Faint are the far ones, coming and going as the sound of bells wafted to a high mountain; loud and clear are the near ones, urgent as an alarm of fire."

Thus is our psychological evolution limited and retarded. But unless we can overcome this difficulty sufficiently to adjust to the imperative demands of new conditions, the issue for civilization is scarcely in doubt.

24

" Modify or disappear " is the inexorable sentence of evolution when the organism is confronted by a changing environment. Man feels the peril of change, and has sought to build breakwaters against the tide by means of written constitutions and printed creeds. The War was but the traditional seventh wave which smashed breakwaters that were already in peril. And in the deluge which accompanied and followed it man has lost confidence. Many things which he imagined were founded on rock he discovered were mainly built on sand.

A curious symptom of the prevailing disillusionment is the turning of the white races to the coloured ones for artistic inspiration : pictures of the South Sea Islanders, carved wooden images from Tahiti, jazz music, negro spirituals. The world resounds with dark laughter as the white man uneasily shifts the burden on his shoulders. Some of the reasons for this disillusionment and loss of confidence are obvious ; others are more deeply-seated. Man's reaction to Nature varies with the control which he feels he has over it.

Recently Man has become rather overawed by the universe in which he finds himself. He can hardly comprehend the vastness and emptiness of the interstellar spaces, or the minuteness of the electrons within the atom. Life trembles, as it were, in a narrow zone between intolerable heat and intensest cold ; if it wavers on either side it ceases to be. It can only exist in association with an atom which holds twelve electrons within its orbit. Staggered by such facts, he is too apt to forget that the most marvellous of all matter is the nerve-cell and that, so far as we know, he possesses the most highly developed system of such cells, whereby he can perceive and interpret the phenomena by which he is surrounded. The astronomer in H. G. Wells's story realized that he was greater than the comet which was presently going to destroy the earth and him with it, because he knew what the comet was going to do and the comet did not.

But man has become much less confident of the control

which reason can exert over his instincts. It required the convulsion of a great war abruptly to remind us that if we had subdued Nature externally, internally, in ourselves, she is as cruel and bloodthirsty as ever. Man has acquired a control over machines without acquiring anything like a corresponding control over himself. He does not even appear to be able to control satisfactorily something he has created for his own convenience—namely currency. He has a fatal aptitude for applying his discoveries to destructive ends. Aviation has been described recently as " the discovery that took the wrong turning ", and that is typical of much.

Evolution always offers a higher and a lower road : to a form which involves an expanding, more complex unit, or to one which degenerates to a lower level, though more consonant with the capacity of its components. The ascidian, reduced to a jelly-like lump clinging to a rock like a piece of sea-weed, still retains vestiges of its vertebrate origin, and its young start off in each generation as hopeful young vertebrates, until the fatal taint of degeneration strikes them. But that is to look at it from our point of view. The ascidian lazily clinging to that rock may be perfectly happy. This is what makes present-day conditions so disturbing. Whole nations which apparently feel unable to maintain the ideals that we regard as the higher ones actually seem to gain a new hope and a new faith by departing from them. The new level is more suited to their evolutionary development, and they are more comfortable in it. Depreciation of ideals, like depreciation of currency, seems to give them a new stability.

In this process no ideal has suffered so severely as that of liberty. Harold Nicolson inquires: " Is national independence so far more important than personal freedom ? That is a question," he went on to say, " which the present generation are unable to answer." It seems to me that a good many nations have already answered it in the affirmative. The segregating species-making impulse has at any rate for the moment the upper hand.

General Smuts recently made a powerful claim for liberty as the foundation of political health and happiness ; whereas in three-fourths of Europe liberty is now regarded as a curse, tyranny as the way of salvation. It may be that the old ideas of liberty were too negative ; it may well be that the population of large areas of the globe are not yet fit for it. We feel it about India, so we need not be surprised if some European countries feel it about themselves. It is certainly the fact that nineteenth century ideas of liberty were too much bound up with a policy of *laisser-faire* which led to social injustice. It is inevitable that the State shall take an increasing part in planning the lives of its individual citizens. In the same way we are learning that in the body the central nervous system exercises some control even over functions which were thought to be entirely autonomous. I reminded you at the outset that in evolution there are two parallel processes at work—increasing division of labour and increasing co-ordination. The evolution of large industries illustrates both of these. Indeed, the division of labour in a large factory has reached such a pitch that in many occupations craftsmanship is dead and the workman has become a robot. It is therefore significant and encouraging to find that a captain of industry, Lord Stamp, should have devoted his presidential address to the British Association to a consideration of the effects of industrial change upon the social organism ; a subject of great importance to the welfare of the state. He pointed out that when the time span of important change was considerably longer than that of the individual human life, we enjoyed the illusion of fixed conditions. Now the time span is much shorter, but our attitude of mind still tends to regard change as the exceptional and rest as the normal, rather than the converse. But these alternative attitudes make all the difference to the accommodating mechanisms we provide. In one case there will be well developed tentacles, grappling irons, anchorages, and all the apparatus of security. In the other society will put on casters and roller bearings, cushions, and all the aids to painless transition. Thus the

written Constitution of the United States, devised for the
" horse and buggy " days, acts as a serious drag on
adaptations to entirely different conditions. A scientific
study of the effects of scientific discovery itself on both
capital and labour is urgently needed in order to render
the change from obsolescent to new methods as smooth as
possible. As Lord Stamp says : " Since man does not live by
bread alone, if a ruthless industrial organization
continually tears up the family from its roots, transferring
it without choice to new surroundings, destroying the
ties of kin, home and social life, of educational and
recreational environment, it is far from ideal. Human
labour can never be indefinitely fluid and transferable
in a society that has a soul above consumption of mere
commodities." He goes on to discuss the factors
determining the optimum conditions of change, pointing
out that a natural increase of population is both the best
shock absorber and safety valve that the community
can possess, and we are faced with the problem that in all
Western industrial countries the population will shortly
become stationary and then will noticeably decline. He
is content to point out the effects of this and does not
indulge in the scolding which we usually have to listen
to when the falling birth-rate comes under discussion.
Looked at broadly, is it not probable that after the
enormous increase of population in the nineteenth century
there should be a lull ? I do not know whether anthro-
pologists are prepared to explain the outburst of fertility
in North-Eastern Europe and Western Asia in the early
centuries A.D. which swept aside all barriers, inundated
the Roman Empire and dissolved it into fragments.
One can only vaguely visualize the enormous pressure of
population that initiated these huge waves of migration.
But they did not continue indefinitely, and the population
of England was neither great nor rapidly increasing in the
days of Queen Elizabeth, which was certainly not an age
of decadence. If our industrial system really depends for
its success upon an increasing number of individuals to
produce an increasing amount for an increasing

population to consume, it is bound to crash sooner or later. Fortunately Lord Stamp leaves us a loophole by saying that the effects of a static population can be mitigated if the *per capita* income is increasing. Because as the parts of the globe inhabitable by the white races fills up, the population will inevitably become static. Whether the present lull is entirely due to contraceptive practices, or whether there is also some fall in natural fertility it is impossible to say ; certainly medical men see plenty of childless parents who ardently desire offspring. Carr-Saunders in his recent book, *World Population*, thinks it likely that the time may soon come when among white people no more children will be born than are desired before conception. One reviewer, horror-struck at such an idea, said this may mean a far more rapid crumbling away even than that in Great Britain at present, whereas for my part I should expect it to solve many of our psychological problems. Anyhow, if that is the natural trend neither threats nor bribes will alter it ; indeed one might point out that if finance were all, the bribes are so paltry that they would only influence the unthinking type of person who would welcome a shilling even if he knew he would have to pay a sovereign for it later on.

It is gratifying at any rate to be told by Lord Stamp that a higher standard of wealth may compensate for a falling population to some extent, for I believe that this higher standard and more settled conditions would lead to the production of more children to enjoy them, and thus with minor fluctuations the balance would be maintained. But how dangerous is prophecy. I am grateful to Mr. J. A. Spender for reminding us of a book entitled *National Life and Character* by Charles Pearson, which was published in 1893. I remember being greatly impressed by it at the time. Looking ahead, Pearson saw the world becoming duller and quieter ; war would only be occasionally resorted to when arbitration had failed, and even then it was possible to hope that it would be conducted without intentional injury to non-combatants, and with the smallest possible damage to private property. There would be socialism of a limited, bureaucratic, and unprogressive sort ; science had done its greatest work, and the future could have no great discoveries in store ; the general tendency would be towards the static and the somnolent, and so on. Such were the views of this learned and experienced man. Yet as Spender says : " If we wished to find a statement, exact in almost every detail of what has not happened in the subsequent forty years we could hardly do better than go to this book. . . . Greater and more sudden changes have come to pass than in any similar period of history. . . . To the Victorian Liberal who thought of liberty and progress as things established beyond possibility of challenge, the state of several great nations in Europe would have seemed like an eruption from the nether regions." Nor is this change incompatible with what I previously said about the influence of the dead hand, for we are experiencing its regressive drag on an age furnished with more powerful weapons of destruction to assist in its atavistic savagery.

I hope I have made clear what seems to me the present dilemma. The first biological stage of a community is held together by taboo and fertility rites ; individuality is at a discount. In the second, individualities develop and the religious trend is towards individual salvation and personal immortality. The increasing tendency towards individualism becomes incompatible with a highly organized state which a complex civilization requires for, as Maudsley said, the social organism of which the individual is an element only exists by some suppression of his purely self-regarding impulses. The evolutionary demand for an enlargement of the unit excites a defensive reaction towards national segregation. To effect this, freedom of trade, freedom of exchange, freedom of intercourse, and personal freedom have to be rigorously suppressed. But although human beings in a community are the equivalent of the cells in an organism, they have achieved self-consciousness and individuality. If therefore the repressing force upon their originating and creative powers is strong enough these powers will die and degeneration will follow. *Laisser-faire* would lead to disintegration, and autocracy would lead to mental and moral slavery. The solution can only be found by a method which gives adequate freedom to the individual life within a larger co-ordinated unit. Can we achieve it? Perhaps we are neither wise enough nor good enough. It is no more reasonable to blame the present epoch for its savage and infantile psychology than it would be to blame the Brontosaurus for its tiny brain. Has this civilization to go back to the melting pot like its predecessors? If so another will rise in its place. Of that we may be sure, though it is little consolation to us or to our children. In the past, when a civilization has fallen, the rise of the next has been a matter not of years, but of centuries, until some new dominant blend could arise. We are therefore naturally concerned to see the civilization of to-day conserved. If I could show the way, I might well claim the position of a beneficent dictator. All I am aiming at is to illustrate the truth of Maudsley's dictum : " The general law of development which governed the process during the unrecorded ages was the same law which is proved to have worked within the short compass of recorded time—namely the law of the more complex and special development at the cost of the more simple and general." In addition I hope I have analysed some of the defects inherent in that process. " The fault, dear Brutus, is in ourselves," rather than in a malignant fate obscurely moving behind the scenes. Can we not hope that by remorselessly stripping off the labels from outworn symbols, by resolutely adopting reality principles, we may before it is too late realize the latent possibilities in human life, and recognize that the springs of happiness come from within? In the willing co-operation of free individuals for the common weal lies the only solution. Is this a contradiction in terms? I believe not. We are members all of one body.

31

" WE HAVE REASON TO THINK . . ." [1]

I doubly appreciate the honour of being asked to give the prizes here to-day. In the first place it emphasizes the association which has lasted so long between my University and your Hospital. We have recently benefited by the munificent bequest of one who was a loyal son of Cambridge and who also served this hospital well—I mean the late Mr. Marmaduke Sheild.

In the second place it emphasizes another association ; that between my hospital of St. Bartholomew's and yours. That we have sent you good men the past and the present attest alike. In the past the name which has perhaps most closely linked our hospitals together is that of John Hunter, who may be said to be the first to regard medicine as a branch of experimental biology. His famous aphorism, " Don't think, try," may have been misinterpreted, but never more sardonically than by a friend of mine, who commented that out of respect to John Hunter the medical profession for more than a century had been trying not to think. And although we realize that Hunter was merely advocating experiment rather than speculation, there is a sting of truth in the comment. A hundred and fifty years ago, the need for the collection of data was paramount ; to-day there is at least an equal need for the data to be assimilated and co-ordinated by careful thinking.

Let us think for a moment of the enormous change that has occurred since the beginning of the nineteenth century in our realization of the nature and position of man. True, the astronomers had already orientated man in

---

[1] An introductory address delivered at St. George's Hospital Medical School, 1st October, 1934.

space but there was no conception of his position in time. The grandfathers of all my contemporaries believed that the world was created in 4004 B.C. The record of the rocks was not correctly deciphered till early in the nineteenth century ; geology proved to be the Rosetta stone for the interpretation of the age of the world. Then came Biology to teach man that he was no special creation but the outcome of a long process of evolution. In these latter days psychology has shown not only that this applies to man's structure, but that there are sub-human strata also in the dark recesses of his mind. Finally the modern physicist is upsetting the orderly Newtonian physics and neat Daltonian chemistry in which we seniors were brought up, until man is beginning to doubt whether there is any substance in the material universe at all. He is being told that even mathematical truth is only a tribute to the innate craving for order in his own mind. He is being thrown back on the old adage *Cogito, ergo sum*. All the more reason then that he should try to think.

It is perhaps a too ambitious task to attempt to describe how man came to think, but it may be of interest to note how widely our approach to this problem differs from the methods followed in the seventeenth century by such a man as John Locke. Natural science has given us an inevitable bias to proceed from the simple to the complex. The scientist of to-day does not start with the human understanding as Locke did, but with the genesis of the nervous system.

For the time being, man seems to have lost his curiosity as to the origin of life. He recognizes that this is a problem beyond him. Fifty years ago it was not so and colloidal jellies dredged from the depths of the sea were eagerly scanned for evidence of the transition from the non-living to the living, while Charlton Bastian attempted to demonstrate spontaneous generation to the International Medical Congress in London in 1881, regardless of the horrified and repeated cries of " *mon Dieu, mon Dieu* " from the lips of the great Pasteur.

But if we are willing to leave the origin of life unexplored, we are the more interested in its manifestations. Amid all the bombardment which atoms receive at the hands of physicists, until we are doubtful of the entity of any element, life remains faithful to its central carbon atom, with its apparently infinite capacity for forming chains and rings. Only with such chains and rings do we find life associated. Another striking characteristic of life, to which Sir Gowland Hopkins recently called attention, is that it alone, in a universe of which the energy is ceaselessly running down, can oppose a dam, as it were, and hold up that energy at a useful level. It cannot reverse the second law of thermodynamics, of course, but it can delay its action. On this globe, at least, we can assert that the one thing which checks the degradation of energy is life. That is one of its proud prerogatives.

Even single-celled organisms, or colonies of such, show a characteristic feature of life in their irritability, in the biological sense, a responsiveness to various stimuli. In the simplest forms of life this chiefly took the form of response to light and to chemical substances, a method of response which we still show. But a subtler method of response was soon evolved when many-celled organisms appeared. The general " responsiveness " of the outer protective coat or skin became specialized in two different types of cells. They were, indeed, the parents of sensory and of neuro-muscular cells. It became necessary for the guidance of the body that such perceptive cells should develop particularly at its front end. Here therefore the organs of special sense appear, by which the animal knows what it is approaching, by which indeed, as Sherington phrased it, the animal carries its immediate future in front of it.

Before long these special cells, which we may now call nerve cells, began to retreat to a more protected position and congregate into the beginnings of a central nervous system, while retaining their connection with the exterior by means of nerve fibres. It is a little difficult to realize

34

that the brain and spinal cord are buried embryonic skin, that it is skin which receives and modified skin which interprets the messages we receive from the outside world.

Although the sensory message can at once evoke a motor reply, as in a simple reflex action, it is the appearance of a new nerve cell—the connector, or association cell—between the sensory and motor units which marks the beginning of a central nervous system, and it is the multiplication of such association cells on which the growth and increasing complexity of the nervous system mainly depends.

The evolution of vertebrates, however, achieved, freed the brain for almost unlimited development. And when some fishes struggled on to the land and became amphibians, its further development was urgently called for, not only to face a new environment, but to restrain automatic movements, which, however appropriate to fishes balancing themselves in water, had become highly inappropriate to land animals in which fins had become limbs. And so we find, hand-in-hand, the development of increased skilled movements and of the inhibition of unsuitable movements. At this stage we meet not only with simple but also with conditioned reflexes. When Pavlov, already famous for his researches on digestion, visited England in 1906 to describe the way in which he could modify the reflexes in his dogs by training, I little realized how far-reaching the influence of those observations would be. May I say, in passing, that he was particularly happy in his selection of his animal—for no animal is so malleable at the hands of man, whether as to structure or as to conduct, as the dog. The cat will condition her own reflexes, but for the dog our prohibitions soon become his inhibitions.

I need not recapitulate Pavlov's well-known experiments, but I would like to emphasize just three points. Firstly the chain of association of ideas in a dog is a short one, not being capable of more than three links, whereas in ourselves with our much greater wealth of association cells, the chain of ideas aroused by, say, a few chords of music may extend almost to infinity. Secondly, if the dog is deliberately given signals difficult for him to discriminate, all his conditioned reflexes become upset and he becomes neurotic. Pavlov maintains that this is due to his being exposed to an excessive demand for internal inhibitions, a cause, one may say, which is responsible for human neuroses also. Thirdly, if the area of inhibitions is spread widely enough, the dog simply goes to sleep. Note the behaviour of your dog at your meal-time if he knows he will not be fed himself, and that your attention will be diverted from him—the series of negations piles up and soon he is fast asleep, till you rise from the table and he wakes at once. When we wish to sleep we cut off as many afferent impulses as we can, and seek darkness—not to mention quiet, if haply we may find it in this generation which seeketh after noise. But nevertheless in darkness and in quiet the long chain of association cells may carry impulse after impulse and we may woo sleep in vain.

I should like to emphasize again the great leap forward which the brain achieved when vertebrates took to the land. In the ancient part of the brain common to fishes and all other vertebrates reside the centres which order the functions of organic life, but in this part are also the centres of emotional expression, such as we deliberately deny to fishes when, for instance, we describe a man as " fish-like ". Of recent years we have learned much of the functions of these basal ganglia from the grotesque and cruel ravages of the epidemic of lethargic encephalitis. Not only did it disorganize the statics of the body, but it often played havoc with the emotions and conduct of the unfortunate victim. And so we discovered how deep down in the brain the emotions and passions resided, and how violent and unrestrained might be their manifestations when cut off from the control of the calmer, more reasoning, newer part. Disease thus confirmed and extended the experimental evidence already obtained.

Clearly the activities of the brain depend largely on the stream of impulses received from the outside world.

Michael Foster recorded a case of a boy who had general cutaneous anæsthesia, who was deaf, and also blind in one eye. His sole tie with the outside world was through the remaining eye, and when this was covered he went to sleep. But the case of Helen Keller shows how adequately the brain can develop even when the avenues of sight and hearing are both closed. She, however, was two years old when she became blind and deaf.

It has been said that nervous impulses tend to run along accustomed channels. Herein lies the value of training and habit, whereby in course of time a particular track is beaten out, as it were, through the tangled jungle of grey matter in the brain. Recall what happened when you learned to ride a bicycle and the painful efforts of will which were necessary but often insufficient to enable you to retain your seat. Then gradually it became easy, and before long you found you could ride without thinking about it ; indeed, you rode better when you were not thinking of how you were doing it and could devote your attention—and much needed attention these days—to where you were going. Much earlier in life you trained yourself (with some assistance it is true) to walk and then to talk, though it is so long ago that you have forgotten how it was done. But you were also trained in some very vital processes before you were born, for you entered the world knowing how to breathe, how to manage your circulation, and how to digest your appropriate diet. Indeed, if you begin to think about such things you interfere with them ; the rhythm of your breathing alters, your pulse may race and your heart palpitate, while undue anxiety about your diet will give you indigestion. Your far-away subhuman ancestors had learned to do such things for you and you have inherited their knowledge which is now so deeply ingrained that it has become instinctive and automatic.

Thus we see that the result of training is that in many matters we can act promptly and skilfully without bothering our thinking capacity, which is thereby set free for higher tasks. The brain may indeed be compared to an office consisting of several storeys. The lowest part is concerned with vital functions ; above this is the cerebellum which is chiefly concerned with maintaining the balance of the body and regulating muscular movements. The storey above this is concerned with the expression of the emotions. The floor above is the sorting department where all the messages received from below are dealt with and sent on to the appropriate departments above where the directors sit, each in their allotted rooms. These are on the surface or *cortex* of the brain. Starting from behind and working forwards we find first the department concerned with vision, in the front portion of which visual memories are carefully and systematically stored for ready reference, like a card index. In front and slightly below this is the central hearing department with similar stores of memories of sounds including spoken words. Coming further forward, neatly arranged on one side of a deep fold in the surface, are the row of offices for receiving the ordinary sensations sorted out from all parts of the body, and facing them on the other side are the corresponding row whence messages ordering or checking movements are sent out. At one end of this row is a special office on the left side only for speech, but this cannot work properly without drawing on the word memories stored up behind. And then in front of all in a spacious office sits the Head of the Firm—the thinking You, with all this complicated and elaborate machinery at your command as you may imagine, although you are really entirely dependent upon it.

Now comes a strange fact. Just under the Chief's office lie two little structures which each receive impressions of smell. Lower animals have their eyes one at each side, so that they are not capable of stereoscopic vision ; they go on all fours so that their projecting nose is their best informant. The more intelligent animals are those which have been able to shorten their noses sufficiently to bring their eyes to look forwards and thus achieve stereoscopic vision, but until the erect posture was adopted our ancestors were more dependent on smell than

38

on sight, as the dog still is. Standing up on two legs, our noses were removed from the ground with its many significant odours and the structures concerned with smelling began to deteriorate. Yet they are still directly connected with the highest centres, and Michael Foster maintained that our mental associations still cluster most thickly around the sense of smell.

Stereoscopic vision leads to the realization of the *shape* of objects and encourages the testing power of touch, and so to the evolution of the hand, a peculiarly human attribute. And with the development of the hand comes the capacity for acquiring skilled movements which enormously increase our range of activities and which in their turn make a demand for increased development of the brain to direct them. This in its turn increases our perceptions ; thus the skilled movements which led to the making and then to the playing of musical instruments finally stimulated the creative activities of the brain so much that a genius like Beethoven could write an entire symphony when he had become too deaf to hear a note of it. " Heard melodies are sweet, but those unheard are sweeter," sang Keats, and the brain once developed by external impulses can still create when deprived of some of them. It would indeed have been more serious for Beethoven if his memories for sounds had gone wrong instead of his apparatus for hearing them. And our hearing memories are much more important for speech than our visual ones, since man could talk for ages before he could write and every individual talks before he can read. But we depend very much for intelligence in general matters on our visual memories. That our word memories are packed in a definite order is seen when a head injury which may entirely destroy the memory of a foreign language leaves the remembrance of the native tongue untouched. For as we might expect, it is always the language learned first that has its memories most securely packed.

There are two sides to a skilled movement—not only the performance of the right movement, but the checking of the wrong ones. For this power to check or inhibit is a very important function of the higher parts of the brain. It lies at the very root of self-control not only in movements but in all thought and conduct.

Thus the central nervous system has to deal both with internal and external relations, to ensure both internal harmony and harmony as far as may be with the outside world. The infant comes into the world well-equipped in the former respect, but very imperfectly in the latter. Its complete helplessness is in sharp contrast with that of many lower animals at birth. And that leads us to contrast instinct with intelligence. A recent writer, H. E. Mellersh, said : " Most of us have no great affection for fishes or lizards or snakes, nor feel anything but intense dislike for that large, grim, silent phylum that comprises the crabs and lobsters, the spiders and scorpions, and all the insects. I have often come away from the insect house at the Zoo with a feeling of real nausea, and wondered what it was that disgusted, depressed, and even half-frightened me. Positively I think it is their slow, reasonless, undivertible intentness. But what is it negatively ? What do they lack ? One might say they lacked a sense of humour, and be stating a rather obvious but still somehow relevant fact. But one probably could not do better than say : they never play."

This division of the forms of life into those that can, and do, play, and those that do not and cannot is, in fact, an important and significant one. Only mammals and birds play—the warm-blooded creatures. And it is the warm-blooded creatures whose lives are by far the least guided by instinct ; there is the significant connection. A German, Karl Groos, was the first to stress and satisfactorily explain this connection. And he did it so well that although his book, *The Play of Animals*, was first published in 1897 it is still not superseded. The insect, it is pointed out by Groos, is marvellously complete with instincts ; it has practically nothing to learn. The mosquito can fly perfectly—and sting perfectly—as soon as it has changed from that eagerly wriggling larva, hanging head-downwards from the surface of the water, and has squeezed out from its sheath and dried its wings ; the bee can build her cells, always hexagonal, can perform the honey-dance to inform her mates of a new store found, all without learning. But with birds and mammals it is different ; the inherited memory is not there, those incredibly specialized brain tracks do not exist. Indeed, it is only with a great effort that we can realize how much of the elementary art of keeping alive we humans have had to learn.

The advantage would seem at first sight to be with those forms of life so well equipped with particular instincts. And yet we all know that the skill of the mammal, his power to reason and to adjust his action finely in an emergency, is an infinitely more useful possession than the most perfect set of particular (but unadaptable) instincts. The only question is : How does the mammal acquire this skill, this power of reasoned and delicate response ?

And the answer is, of course, play. So Karl Groos, with much detail, pointed out, He called play an instinct in itself—one *generalized* instinct in substitution for a great number of particular ones. He showed in strict Darwinian fashion how the possession of such a generalized instinct would have a " survival value ". If you have acquired no complete set of cut-and-dried answers to the problems of life, but only a single urge to find out the answers for yourself, then you have set a premium at once upon intelligence. And since intelligence is, without question, Nature's most powerful weapon for progress, those who use intelligence will win the race from those who do not.

Karl Groos quotes innumerable examples to prove his point that play is for the young an instinct—is, that is to say, a definite urge. And what is play ? It is mimicry and make-believe. It is, biologically speaking, a practice of powers that have appeared in a crude form early in life, so that when they are needed later thay may already be near perfection. It is not enough for the grown animal to have the simple and unelaborated instinct to fight or to fly in an emergency ; he must have practised those responses assiduously. The necessity for mimicry, there-fore—mimicry of one's elders—is obvious. But the need for make-believe is essential too. For the real situation either will not or cannot be allowed to arrive in youth. The kitten must needs be able to pretend to itself that the paper is the live mouse before it can acquire the skill to catch one ; the hare must learn to be fleet and nimble without a real carnivore after it every time. And so we begin to see how the enormous power to make-believe arrives in us humans. It has again a " survival value " ; it is a part of us, it is a fundamental instinct. Our theatre and our arts come (via the meetings and ceremonies and solemn dances of primitive man) from this manifestation of mammal's necessary urge to play.

And though that is an old story, perhaps it has not been pondered upon quite enough. Karl Groos pondered upon it further, and came to the conclusion that there was an added inducement to make-believe in the " freedom " that it gave. In real life we are too often the playthings of the opposing forces about us. But in make-believe it is ourselves who are always the masters, who *make things happen*. Life, in fact, is too real—and so play is earnest. All of us—all of us warm-blooded animals—love to feel that we are the prime movers of something, however trivial ; we love to " work our own sweet will ". We all (as the psychologists say now) love to exert the power instinct.

Man loves to play and make-believe through all his life ; there we are different from the other mammals who do not seem much driven by the play-instinct once they are grown up. It is the birds who, besides ourselves, play most when they are no longer young. And it is the birds who are excitable creatures, have a blood heat even above our own, and have another element and another dimension in which to sport.

And yet man is the supreme grown-up play addict. The urge has, in fact, become most elaborated in him, the most elaborated creation. It may be caused by many

42

desires, seemingly contradictory, but all arising from that original generalized instinct of the warm-blooded. We may play from a desire to practice and " keep fit ", from a desire to turn from difficult reality to pleasant make-believe, a desire to exercise power and skill, a desire for excitement, a desire to achieve thrills. And here we may recall Keith's saying that man of all animals has retained the power to carry on youthful characteristics into adult life. He may indeed carry them too far, as I thought when a man of 45 told me that the one thing he lived for was to lower his handicap at golf !

But intelligence and accurate perception, however necessary to thought, do not themselves constitute thought. If Socrates discoursing with Phædrus on the banks of the Ilissus could not define thought, neither can I be expected to do so. But I like Rodin's sculptured vision of " Le Penseur ". At first sight that low-browed squatting figure, brooding with chin resting on knuckle, hardly seems to typify thought, until one realizes that it represents the dawn of thought, the painful gestation of ideas in the caveman's mind. At what stage precisely do the twin streams of temperament arising from the internal afferent impulses and of perceptions from the outside world, ascending through chains of association cells enriched by experience, attain in the highest levels of the brain to the dignity of abstract thought ?

You will, I hope, forgive me if I am attempting a biological rather than a metaphysical approach to a problem I am not prepared to solve. For I do believe that this method has in comparatively few years carried us further towards a comprehension of the workings of man's mind than centuries of metaphysics have achieved. As Robert Bridges said : " Man's Reason is in such deep insolvency to sense " that

> " Not without alliance of the animal senses
> Hath she any miracle."

One may fairly say that one of the most recent

achievements of man's reason is his recognition of how unreasonable a being he is. To quote the same poet—
" How small a part of Universal Mind can conscient Reason
    claim !
  'Tis to the unconscious mind as the habitable crust is to
    the mass of the earth."

But this narrow crust of reason has a great, and as Rodin saw, a painful task. It has to co-ordinate here and repress there these streams of afferent impulses which pouring through the basal ganglia have gained in turbulence and in turbidity by stirring emotional depths inherited from long dead ancestors as well as those acquired in earlier life. It is no light task to provide for the precipitation of the mud, for the clarification of the streams and, to pursue the simile, usefully to employ them to irrigate the higher centres for the fertilization of thought. Perhaps, as Adler says, nothing is quite so conscious and nothing quite so unconscious as we imagine. Indeed the frontier is an indefinite and changing one. But reason properly used will agree to recognize the place that the emotions should be accorded in life. It is perhaps due to mental attitudes in the past which tended to exaggerate the rôle of reason that there has arisen an undoubted and undue depreciation of reason in these latter days. For whole nations politics have become total abandonment of the right of judgment into the hands of a dictator, while a religious movement of the day relegates the individual conscience to the guidance of a group. I do not intend to discuss either politics or religion. I merely wish to illustrate how widespread is the individual's lack of confidence to-day in his own power of reason. But perhaps the process can be best observed in certain literary movements which, starting with an angry reaction against the intellect, such as D. H. Lawrence, for instance, displayed, has gradually deteriorated into what appears to me to be mere baby talk. Whatever this may mean to the writer himself—or herself, I must add, since Gertrude Stein is one of the most notorious exponents of the " cocky-locky, henny-penny " style of writing which was formerly reserved for the delectation of the nursery—it can, from the nature of the case, communicate very little to anyone who does not possess the key. That inspiration wells up from the unconscious, or at least the subconscious, would be generally admitted, but just as the highest level of the brain selects the sensory impressions to which it will pay attention, so reason must arrange and select the messages from the emotional levels. To-day only too often a writer fishes up from the unconscious what appears to him to be a pearl worthy to be treasured, but which seems to the onlooker nothing but a worthless pebble. Why are other people's dreams so utterly boring to everyone except a psycho-analyst? Because the narrator cannot reproduce the emotional affect which accompanied the dream. The artist by judicious and intellectual arrangement of the material derived from this inspiration may be able to convey the thrill, but the writers against whom I am protesting persist in hurling the crude material at one in raw slabs. Another barrier to comprehension they raise is this. On the way up from the deeper layers an impulse may run through a series of association cells, stimulating memories which are entirely individual to the person who experiences them. If he flings those associated ideas at us without a clue, he is really speaking in a foreign language. Although this method is used even in prose it is, of course, more frequently employed in what is called modern poetry. Mr. T. S. Eliot, for instance, who is bleakly austere in prose says that in poetry meaning only plays the part of the lump of meat in the turned-up end of the dog-stealer's trousers. Meaning is only required to focus the reader's attention until the poem has him in thrall. Well that may be so, but I still hanker after that bit of meat when I read an alleged poem like this :—

> If it was to be a prize a surprise
> if it was to be a surprise to realize,
> if it was to be if it were to be, was it to be.
> What was it to be. It was to be what it was.

And it was. So it was. As it was. As it is.
As it as it is. It is and as it is and as it is.
And so and so as it was.
Keep it in sight all right.

" Milton, thou should'st be living at this hour.
England hath need of thee."

It is interesting to recall, by the way, that a tendency
to link words together by sound rather than by meaning
is a reversion to an infantile mode. The repetition of such
sounds is attributed to the control over the speech not
being as yet completely developed. It is shown in the
first words the child speaks " Mamma, Papa, Nana ",
and this kind of repetition is to be noted in the stories
which delight very young children. It is therefore not
without significance that one of the new artistic movements christened itself " Dada ".

And as to prose, what is one to make of this extract
from James Joyce's latest lucubration ?

" The flossies all and the mossies all they drooped
upon her draped brimfall. The bowknots, the showlots,
they wilted into woeblots. The pearlagraph, the pearlagraph, knew whitchly whether to weep or laugh. For
always down in Carolinas lovely Dinahs vaunt their
views."

This is bad enough, but it is even more serious when a
critic tells us that this is slapstick raised to the status of
art, and that the delight which one finds in such words is
sharper than the ordinary pleasure of prose. Surely it
is time, in the name of reason, to challenge this pretentious high-brow nonsense and to call its bluff.

Well the more youthful members of my audience may
say, how can you expect to appreciate the new beauties
that are being revealed by these modern writers. You
are so hardened by established conventions and outworn
modes that naturally you are deaf to this new music.
Very well, then let me ask you to listen to the views of
Mr. John Sparrow, an eminent but quite youthful critic.
His recent book, *Sense and Poetry*, is a devastating criticism
of this new school. May I quote a few passages—" We

46

are now to be told that . . . experience, hitherto taken to be the raw material of art, should be accepted as its finished product. . . . One of the chief reasons for the unintelligibility of modern verse is the predominance of associations that are personal to the writer. Egoism is carried so far that poems are written for the appreciation of which a complete account of their author's external and internal life is needed. . . . Those who write unintelligible poetry . . . find themselves justified by the beliefs of an increasingly popular school of thought which in effect denies the existence of the intellect. . . . To make the fullest use of the associative value both of words and of what words stand for has been the task of literature since literature was first attempted. . . . Modern writers therefore do not break new ground in paying attention to the effects of association ; what is new in their writing is the result of their paying attention to association alone and exploring it so thoroughly that meaning is entirely or almost entirely superseded." Or as Mr. Desmond MacCarthy says, it is hopeless to reproduce in print the very texture of consciousness, such as leads Mr. James Joyce to record the jabberings of the idiot or flat-headed savage who talks unheard in the backward abyss of our minds and sometimes screams audibly in delirium. Mr. Sparrow has clearly defined the symptoms, but as medical men we want to go behind the symptoms and determine the causes at work, here as elsewhere. Mr. Gerald Heard, in his recent book *These Hurrying Years*, has attempted this task. He attributes them to a growth in self-consciousness, a new realization of what the mind is doing. While this development has seemed to many onlookers only " the treason of the clerks ", the betrayal of reason, the blind escape into childishness, superstition and self comforting illusion, he does not so regard it. What we have to focus upon is the force, the cause which has produced that reaction. He thinks that we need not be unduly per- turbed by the new experiments, since they are all part of a growth which though largely blind to-day, is making

47

for a new synthesis. He admits that this may be too optimistic, and I think it is clear that the pendulum has swung too far. I have great belief in the capacity of life to adapt itself to its environment. But of one thing I am sure, we shall never achieve a new civilization by denying reason its place. Even though we realize that it does not include the whole of life, it must have the final word. To quote a saying of Gaskell's which will bear repetition—" The race is not to the swift, nor to the strong, but to the wise."

When I was seeking for a title to express the viewpoint to which I wished to direct your attention, I remembered an essay by that charming writer, Stephen Paget, in which he said:

" Great words and phrases [may] come down in the world. For instance, I have reason to believe— a phrase of noble birth and of the utmost refinement— is at the mercy of gossip. I have reason to believe that the conductor gave me sixpence short on purpose ; and so forth. Quick, let us do honour to this old phrase —for it is descended from two of the stateliest of all words." It occurred to me to adapt that phrase, hoping thus to make a plea for the restoration of reason to its throne on the highest level of the nervous system—the last to come, the first to go, but all the more to be cherished on that account ; reason is the judge and assessor of our instincts and our emotions which, however necessary for driving energy, if uncontrolled are but blind leaders of the blind. We have reason by which to think . . .

THE RETURN TO ÆSCULAPIUS [1]

Science builds up steadily on the foundations already laid down ; art is more at the mercy of changing fashion. Indeed, to-day many of the arts seem anxious to disregard tradition altogether ; but medicine, while becoming increasingly scientific, must remain always largely an art, and one which must be scrupulous to retain such traditions as are of proved value and of good report. And as I think of the marriage of science to art in medicine, the vision rises before my eyes of the Ionian Sea. We had sailed from Athens and passed Sunium, where the marble columns of the temple still shine in the sun, marking the point at which the homeward-bound Athenian is reputed to have caught the first glimpse of the glittering spear held by the statue of Pallas Athene on the Acropolis. We had threaded between many islands, and just before we reached Rhodes another island arose, blue cliffs out of a deep blue sea. It was Cos, the cradle of medical science. Here, under the fostering care of Hippocrates, temple ritual was invaded by the methods of the medical school. Magic was replaced by observation. Disease was no longer regarded as the work of evil spirits or the results of spells cast from without, but as the logical outcome of disturbed natural processes. But in spite of that revolutionary idea which replaced the priest by the physician, man is all too prone to look back, longing to return to the past, with its ritual and magic.

In *Marius the Epicurean* Walter Pater gave a vivid

[1] Based on an address from the chair of the Medical Society of Individual Psychology, 15th October, 1931, and on the Sir Charles Hasting's Memorial Lecture at the British Medical Association.

account of a visit to a Roman temple of Æsculapius when Marius was a boy.

" The evening came as they passed along a steep white road with many windings among the pines, and it was night when they reached the temple, the lights of which shone out upon them as they paused before the gates of the sacred enclosure, and Marius became alive to a singular purity in the air. A rippling of water about the place was the only thing audible as they waited till two priestly figures, speaking Greek to each other, admitted them into a large, white-walled, and clearly lighted guest-chamber, in which, as he partook of a simple but wholesomely prepared supper, Marius still seemed to feel pleasantly the height they had attained to among the hills.

" The agreeable sense of all that was spoiled by only one thing, his old fear of serpents ; for it was under the form of a serpent that Æsculapius had come to Rome ; and the last definite thought of his weary head before he fell asleep had been a dread either that the god might appear, as he was said sometimes to do, under this hideous aspect, or perhaps one of those great sallow-hued snakes themselves, kept in the sacred place, as he had also heard was usual.

" After an hour's feverish dreaming he woke—with a cry, it would seem, for someone had entered the room with a light, but the footsteps of the youthful figure which approached and sat by his bedside were certainly real. Ever afterwards when the thought arose in his mind of some unexpected but entire relief from distress, like blue sky in a storm at sea, would come back the memory of that gracious countenance which, amid all the kindness of its gaze, had yet a certain air of dominance over him so that he seemed now for the first time to have found the master of his spirit."

Evidently Marius at once acquired a positive trans-ference, as Freud would call it, which would add effect to the discourse of psychological explanation which followed. And then Pater continues : " When he awoke again in that exceeding freshness which he had felt on his arrival the evening before, but with the clear sunlight all about him, it seemed as if his sickness had really departed with the terror of the night ; a confusion had passed from the brain, a painful dryness from the hands. It was a delight merely to be alive and there." Which I take to be a true picture of the sense of release which comes to the psychoneurotic when a complex is resolved. He goes on to discuss very beautifully the life within the precincts, but not in such terms as would help our present purpose ; for that we must turn to other sources of information.

Curiously enough one of the most vivid accounts is that given in a satirical vein by Aristophanes in the " Plautos " when Plautos goes to be cured of his blindness. " First we took him to the water and then gave him a bath. . . . Then we went to the precinct of the god. When our wafers were laid on the altar, the preparatory sacrifices made, and our cake in the flame of Hephaistos, we laid Plautos down on a couch and we all put straight our mattresses. . . . When the servant of the god put out the lamps and told us to go to sleep and keep silent if we heard a noise, all of us lay down quickly." He describes how the god appeared and went round examining the ailments in turn. . . . " Thereafter he sat down by Plautos and first touched his head ; and then took a clean towel and wiped his eyelids. Panakeia (the daughter of Æsculapius) wrapped his head and all his face in a purple cloth. Then the god whistled, and two serpents of prodigious size rushed out from the temple. Then these two crept gently under the purple cloth and licked his eyelids round about. And before you could drink ten measures of wine, Plautos stood up, a seeing man." One can well believe that a functional disorder might be cured by such a drastic treatment by suggestion, when the mind had been prepared by the rites. It is curious how man's primitive fear of serpents was turned to therapeutic purpose. The serpent in the wilderness is an outstanding example of this.

Cawadias takes the view that the medical art was not practised during the first few centuries of the temple's prosperity. The earlier methods were rendered impossible in course of time by the rapid growth of scepticism. People refused to believe in miracles and new methods had to be devised if the temple was to be carried on by medical science and hygienic treatment, while for evident reasons the cult had to be preserved. Thus we find a combination of therapeutics and religious worship. As Mary Hamilton shows, the treatment is still by temple sleep, but now the god does not save by personal action. He points out the way to salvation. Dreams were sent and token given to the suppliant and an interpretation of these had to be made. According to the interpretation the patient pursued what seems to have been a long and tedious process of cure. Such treatment necessitated lengthy residence at the temple, so that it became a kind of hydropathic establishment whither crowds flocked in search of health.

To the success of the treatment which in itself was hygienic, the healthy situation of the temple and the health-giving waters of the sacred well would largely contribute. To this day the belief in the health-giving waters of the sacred well persists, and invalids flock in crowds to spas to drink of waters that are often nauseous unless plentifully flavoured by faith. They attribute to these waters the benefit they derive from a pleasant holiday in a healthy place, aided by massage, electricity, and medical skill. The ordinary hygienic measures ordained by Æsculapius were cold bathing, bleeding, anointing with mud or sand, walking with bare feet, exercise in the open air, and riding. The medicinal remedies were various and curious. Sometimes operations were carried out under the influence of hypnotism. The discovery of a number of Steles at Epidauros in 1885 has given us a clear record of the methods practised. Thus on one we read: " A man had an abdominal abscess. He saw a vision, and thought that the god ordered the slaves who accompanied him to lift him up and hold him, so that his abdomen could be cut open. The man tried to get away, but his slaves caught him and bound him. So Æsculapius cut him open, ridding him of the abscess, and then stitched him up again, releasing him from his bonds. Straightway he departed cured and the floor of the Abaton was covered with blood." Evidently here hypnosis was used as a partial and not altogether successful anæsthetic. Fortunately the operation was successful. But a very important part of the treatment was the interpretation of dreams by priests which was accepted as a divine inspiration. From this developed a more or less definite psychotherapy.

Cleanliness, fresh air, dream analysis, and psychological explanation ; these, I repeat, were the cardinal tenets of the Æsculapian cult, and it is a striking fact that all of them were lost by medicine until quite recent times. The bathroom was an almost unknown adjunct to a private house until about 1860. Fresh air was anathema for the sick until about the beginning of the present century. Prior to that, night air was imagined to be fraught with deadly perils. The patient with a delicate chest had every breath of fresh air carefully excluded from his room, and when he walked abroad he was muzzled with a black gag, most inappropriately termed a respirator. Until the war psychotherapy was looked upon as a crank and studiously avoided by the majority of the medical profession as savouring of quackery. To-day we have returned to the cult of Æsculapius and are his faithful disciples But the history of his cult provides us with an interesting example first of the making of a god, and then of the replacement of his magical methods by lay medicine. Is not this the whole history of therapeutics ? Organotherapy sprang from the crude sympathetic magic, and the savage warrior ate the heart of his foe to acquire his bravery and strength. To quote Dr. Charles Singer—" The overwhelming mass of earlier Greek medical literature sets forth for us a pure scientific effort to observe and to classify disease, to make generalizations from carefully collected data, to explain the origin of disease on rational grounds and to apply remedies when possible on a reasoned basis." But: " There is ample evidence that the Greeks inherited, in common with many other peoples of the Mediterranean and Asiatic origin, a whole system of magical or at least non-rational pharmacy and medicine from a remoter ancestry." Thus: " It is interesting to connect the Æsculapian snake cult with the prominence of the serpent in Minoan religion." And again: "The extreme cult of prognosis among the Coans may not improbably be traced back to the medical lore of the temple soothsayers."

It has been suggested to me that the rapid rise of Greek medicine was due to the fact that there was a considerable body of Sumerian medicine which has subsequently become decadent, but being still in existence, was capable of revival. In this connection I would call your attention to an interesting analysis of the first four chapters of the Book of Daniel by Dr. James, who regards the description of the illness of Nebuchadnezzar as a skilful pen-picture of a maniac-depressive temperament, and Daniel as a fine type of civil servant who was also a resourceful psychiatrist.

Be that as it may, by 500 B.C. Alcmæon had insisted on the doctrine " health depends upon harmony, disease upon discord of the elements within the body ". This, however inadequately achieved, was the aim of the Æsculapian cult. In our own day the development of scientific medicine did for a time divert attention from the patient as an individual. The rise of morbid anatomy, bacteriology, and bio-chemistry in turn tended to this. But medicine is a department of biology and unless we consider the patient as a whole, as a living organism reacting to changes in either the external or the internal environment, we shall miss an essential part of his case. Ordinary materialistic medicine is apt to forget the fact that the patient's emotional and mental outlook will inevitably influence, and be influenced by his disease ; the psychotherapist is apt to forget that the patient has a body which may be suffering from some physical distress.

There was much in the temple ritual which may seem like quackery to-day, but I would prefer to call it psychotherapy adapted to the needs of those times. To-day there is still a craving for magical cures ; the common phrase " it worked like magic " expresses that deep if subconscious desire. After all, our reason is a much more recent acquisition than our emotions. Our forefathers for many thousands of years depended for healing on magic alone ; even the first approaches to rational medicine are as yesterday compared with the reign of magic. That alone would suffice to make the appeal of the quack the more powerful, for he appeals to an incredibly old Adam who claims many descendants. And when health is shaken it is the most recently acquired, the highest levels of the central nervous system, that most easily lose control, and the primitive man peeps out of the cave in which reason has shamefacedly tried to conceal him.

In addition to a craving for magic there is another tendency which affects us all ; to seek security in authority. There are some things about which it is too painful to be in doubt. Certainty is sought in authority, without too critical an inquiry into the source of that authority. This tendency has repeatedly asserted itself in the history of medicine and has frequently delayed its progress. The authority of Aristotle, Galen, and the Church have each in their own way been detrimental in this respect. Whereas Hippocrates placed reliance on general methods, Galen exalted the importance of drugs, a fact of which the term " Galenicals " still reminds us. Galen departed from the simplicity of Hippocrates and evolved such subtle and complicated theories, such definite and artificial classifications that the original doctrines were almost lost sight of, especially in therapeutics. Not only so, but the medieval mentality, always subservient to authority, elevated Galen's writings to the level of papal infallibility, to question which was blasphemy. Only among the Arabs and at Salerno in Italy was the torch kept feebly burning. It required the sceptical inquiring mind of the Renaissance, the rebirth of the Greek spirit, in fact, to fan that torch into flame again.

The craving for magic and authority which is inherent in us all, especially when we are ill, has undoubtedly helped the doctor in the treatment of his patient. The gold-headed cane of the physician of the past became his rod of Æsculapius and when he cast it aside and tried to appeal to rational and scientific procedures he lost a powerful weapon. In no other way can I account for the fact that at a time when medical science has been advancing at a rate previously unknown, there is more scepticism and doubt as to the value of the services we render than ever before. Our patients may like us as individuals, but as a profession we have a " bad press ".

It is worth while to consider some of the causes of the grievous misunderstandings between those who desire restoration of health and those who sincerely wish to help them to achieve it. For no one who has lived among doctors can doubt that they are filled with a genuine zeal for healing.

No one is entirely rational and everyone when ill is less rational than usual. The late Dr. Gee told me that once Sir William Gull was descanting at dinner on his favourite topic that the successful medical man must be a bit of a quack. It is the old story, he said, *plebs vult decipi*. Dr. Martin promptly translated this as " the public like to be gulled ", but his witticism was not appreciated by Sir William. I would prefer to put it that the quack obtains his success by unintelligent and often dishonest psychotherapy. He can only be defeated by psychotherapy that is both intelligent and honest. The quack uses both authority and magic. He adopts an air of infallibility which is impressive but unwarranted. A doctor with his knowledge of the limitations of his art cannot honestly assume that air. A quack seizes on the latest scientific discovery and turns it to magical ends.

We have seen hypnotism, electricity, radium, and light each in turn exploited in this way, and I was not surprised lately to hear of a quack who purported to cure by cosmic rays. The patient knows that each of these discoveries has scientific sanction and is therefore favourably disposed towards their therapeutic use. He thinks the orthodox profession is too conservative to accept them, and he does not realize that any agency powerful enough to have a beneficial effect can also have a harmful one if unskilfully or ignorantly employed.

But there is another reason for the appeal that quackery makes and one less creditable to our profession. Medicine is an enormous field to cover and I would assert that every successful form of unorthodox practice owes its success to neglect of some part of that field by us. The bonesetter owes his success to the disregard of manipulative surgery in the past; the homœopath to our former failure to apply expectant treatment. Expectant treatment does not mean " wait and see ", it means following the natural course of the disease, ready to help nature at the appropriate moment, ready to relieve symptoms as they arise. It involves care that our remedies should not do harm. The homœopath at least uses remedies that can not do harm and he waits upon the *vis medicatrix naturae*. But he asserts as a generalization that like cures like, and maintains that anyone who does not accept this generalization must believe that unlike cures unlike, and labels him an allopath. This is as logical as a man asserting that the moon is made of green cheese, and when we deny it, labelling us as chalkites on the strength of the saying " as different as chalk from cheese ". If we do not believe it is one, it must be the other. We accept no such generalizations ; we study the reactions of the individual to the invasions of disease and are prepared to adopt any means that offer reasonable expectation of helping the patient.

I have said before, and despite the protests I then received, I repeat that the great defect of homœopathy is that Hahnemann's conceptions, though in some respects progressive at the time he enunciated them, have been crystallized into a creed by his disciples. Many ideas in orthodox medicine originated from no more reasonable grounds than Hahnemann's but we are free to cast these aside and we do so as knowledge progresses. Similarly Christian Science owed its rise to the fact that pre-War medicine was far too materialistic. We did not allow sufficiently for the influence of the mind upon the body. But Christian Science while recognizing this merely meets it by suggesting that the cause of a mental distress does not exist ; it makes no attempt to bring the cause of such distress into consciousness, thus enabling it to be dealt with. It may confer a temporary passive immunity, as it were, but it cannot confer an active immunity which enables the mind to deal with the trouble in the many forms which a psychoneurosis, like a chameleon, may assume.

But a cult which to-day is raising a threatening head against the whole body of natural science is osteopathy. There is gross misconception on this subject. Most laymen with whom I have discussed the subject have been under the impression that it is merely a grander name for bonesetting, which is far from being the case.

I may well be challenged to explain the successes of osteopaths. Eliminating, as one must in fairness, the cases of hysterical conditions which would be cured by any method of treatment sufficiently impressive, there remain cases which are amenable to skilful manipulative treatment. We must distinguish between osteopathy as a craft and as a theory of disease. As a craft it can conceivably be useful if the diagnosis has been made by a fully trained and qualified man. There are qualified surgeons who have studied osteopathic methods of treatment, who accept its limitations and, most important of all, know when not to use it. Most of us could relate grim tales of the disasters following its use in unsuitable cases.

But if the theory of osteopathy is right then the whole body of scientific evidence that has been laboriously built up during the last hundred years or so by workers all over the civilized world, is wrong, root and branch. Are you prepared to make such a sweeping assertion?

I might say in answer to the gibe so often made that the profession has at first rejected doctrines which subsequently proved to be correct, that if some truths have been so rejected it does not follow that the doctrines we reject are necessarily true. Yet that attitude is implied by the rejected in medicine, in art, and in literature alike.

Another source of misunderstanding, and a very fertile one, is that patient and doctor do not speak the same language. The patient seeketh after a label and for a cause. Yet the label cannot convey much to the mind of someone who has not been through an elaborate training, and a training which has taught him that the cause of many diseases is unknown.

Sir Farquhar Buzzard dealt with this aspect in his Maudsley Lecture with his accustomed clarity and good sense. He said: "The man in the street is familiar enough with the term ' scientific research ', but has little conception of how scientific observations are registered and controlled, how deductions are tested and hypotheses scrapped. He lives in another world, and is content to welcome a ' new discovery ', sensational enough to attract notice in the press, as a bolt from the blue, or as a species of miracle, and to accept it without interest in its origin, its evolution, or the authority on which it is proclaimed." Sir Farquhar's remedy for this difficulty is not " to bring the layman, totally unprepared, face to face with the spectre of disease through the agency of lectures, of the press, or of the wireless ", but to make biology, the science of life, part of general education. Everyone should know something of the nature and facts of life before taking on its responsibilities. He went on to say: " To observe, follow, and appreciate the scrupulous precision and cautious control of any scientific inquiry would not only engender an early and enduring relish for Nature's verities, but avoid the flagrant and pathetic credulity so characteristic of those who have had no such education. Further, a more general desire to seek after truth, and a greater disinclination to accept statements from all kinds of sources at their face value, would be of immense advantage to the future of civilization as a whole, quite apart from the effect on the practice of medicine." I would suggest an additional argument for the study of biology. This is an age of machines and we are becoming machine-minded. People who know every detail of a motor car may know nothing of physiology, and so come to think of their bodily mechanism in terms of engines—a very false analogy. Incidentally this makes them more impatient with the doctor who cannot supply a spare part, and who forbears to remind them that a motor car is often scrapped.

Another cause of our unpopularity as a profession is the mistaken idea the public have of the canons of medical etiquette, which they regard as an awesome mystery. As I told a distinguished luminary of the church who wished me to treat him behind his doctor's back, medical etiquette is merely the application of the golden rule, do unto others as you would they should do unto you. This I said, knowing that I should see his face no more. Yet it is true. Just as we are genuinely anxious to treat our patient honestly and do our best for him, so we act towards our colleague in the belief that he is similarly actuated. If the patient will put himself in the position of trying to do his best for someone and consider how he would wish others to behave to him while so doing, his own good feeling should solve for him all questions of medical etiquette.

It is curious that it was just during the most materialistic phase of medicine that scepticism as to the efficacy of drugs was most rife. The discovery that the body itself manufactured drugs, as it were, such as thyroxin, adrenalin, pituitrin, and insulin, restored the belief that it could be influenced by chemical means. The discovery of vitamins proved how infinitesimal the dose of such chemical substances need be. The discovery that many drugs act by facilitating or checking the entrance into the tissue of the chemical substance liberated by nervous stimuli, opens out a new vista of what one may call natural pharmacology. Our drug treatment must aim at assisting as far as possible the chemical reactions of which the body is the laboratory. Another thing which has been realized is the importance of the effective dose. This we have learned from a study of the anæmias, which has shown that both liver and iron are useless unless a certain dosage is adopted, at which level benefit rapidly ensues. Insulin also has taught us the paramount importance of adjusting our dosage to metabolic requirements. With these new developments in scientific pharmacology, we can have a more assured confidence in influencing the body by chemical means and the fashion of agnosticism on that subject till recently prevalent may well now vanish.

But that drugs are not the whole of medicine, the modern return to Æsculapius testifies in the development of psychotherapy. Psychology was for long a purely academic study, allied to philosophy and metaphysics. It was studied merely by the method of introspection. Then Wundt developed the experimental method which in a way was the extension of the study of the special senses, concerning itself with the mechanism of perception, and not merely of reception, of stimuli. Finally a breach in the great wall of psychology was made by medical men and the whole subject was transformed, while the influence on medicine has been profound. The individual patient again begins to count for something. As Dr. Bernard Hart has said : " He was no longer regarded as ' the uninteresting vehicle of a fascinating disease process '. " The dualism of mind and body has broken down under the assaults of psychologically minded physicians and disease and unhappiness alike can be seen as the resultant of forces in the individual and his environment. The psychiatrist and biochemist can find a common meeting ground in the fact that all nervous mechanisms produce their effect through the intermediary of chemical substances. This new synthesis of mind and body, this conception of the individual as a dynamic entity is the outstanding achievement of twentieth century medicine and will greatly influence its future.

For me the significance of this modern return to Æsculapius is the recognition of the importance not only of the disease which the patient has, but of the patient which has the disease ; his reactions as an individual, his environment, and his hereditary trends. The old adage " examine the whole of your patient " thus assumes a new meaning. It is by this combined attack on the physical and psychological side that medicine in the future will make advance and still further aid human suffering.

Macfie Campbell says : " The mechanism by which [man] adapts himself to the simpler factors in the environment have been made the object of intensive study, and medicine can claim that it has increased the number of infants who survive and has prolonged the span of individual life. So far medicine has given scant consideration to the mechanism by which man adapts himself to the social environment. . . ." " The medical profession now boasts proudly of the quantitative addition it has made to human life ; the time may come when it will point out with equal pride to measures which have added to the quality of human life, and have helped the individual and the group to deal more sanely and soundly with those vital issues upon the management of which the special significance and value of human life depend."

I should like at this point to bear testimony to the work of W. H. R. Rivers, whose loss we must still deplore. In my opinion few were so well equipped to lay the foundations of a sane psychotherapy for few psycho-therapists had his biological training.

Soon after the War I picked up a copy of Siegfried Sassoon's new poems in Rivers's rooms at Cambridge and read the one entitled, " To a very wise man." Turning to the title-page I found it endorsed in the author's handwriting with the same phrase, and thus I learned what Rivers's help had meant to him of which he has now told the whole story in *Sherston's Progress*. I got to know Rivers very well when he became a Fellow Commoner at St. John's. In those days he was very reserved in mixed company, and was hampered by a stammer which he had not yet entirely overcome. But if among two or three friends his conversation was full of interest and illumination. He was always out to elicit the truth, entirely sincere, and disdainful of mere dialectic. In the laboratory he devoted himself to experimental psychology of the Wundt type. In 1897 I got him to come and address the Abernethian Society at St. Bartholomew's Hospital. The occasion was not an unqualified success. He chose " Fatigue " as his subject, and before he had finished his title was writ large on the faces of his audience. He had not yet acquired the art of expressing his original ideas in an attractive form except in private conversation.

In 1898 an event occurred which was not only a turning point in his own career, but which was also fraught with far-reaching consequences to English medicine. Yet it was not initiated by a medical man at all, but by an anthropologist, A. C. Haddon, who organized an expedition to the Torres Straits, and took Rivers, William McDougall, and C. S. Myers with him. They went as physiologists ; they returned as psychologists. This was in effect the beginning of the new psychology in England. McDougall's work in this respect has been accorded a wide and popular recognition. Myers has placed the study of industrial fatigue on a scientific basis. Rivers went specially to investigate the vision of uncivilized peoples. He came to the conclusion that while no substantial difference exists between the visual acuity of civilized and uncivilized peoples, the latter show a definite lack of colour discrimination. I believe that the Homeric poems show a similar lack. This suggests that much of colour perception is central rather than peripheral, psychological rather than physiological. It was extraordinarily fascinating to me to watch the evolution of Rivers from a physiologist, particularly concerned with the special senses, into an anthropologist, with a shrewd insight into the mentality of savages, based on a study of their sensory discrimination, and then into a psychotherapist.

He applied and extended Hughlings Jackson's great generalization of the three levels of the central nervous system in a remarkable way to explain certain mental processes. As is well known Hughlings Jackson regarded these three levels—reflex, sensori-motor, and psychical— as representing successive stages in the development of the central nervous system, and maintained that in the disintegrative process of disease the highest, most recently acquired levels were the ones which would suffer first. Many symptoms of nervous disease were due to uncontrolled action of lower levels released from the restraint of higher levels. Rivers extended this conception by postulating a number of different layers, as it were, within the highest level. The development of the individual mind led to the formation of consecutive layers, each possessed of more reality-principle and self-control. But each individual started out equipped in these lower layers with earlier racial tendencies which were held more or less in abeyance by the higher layers. One might compare this part of the brain to that deep cleft in the rocks near Garavan, where for 100,000 years men dwelt, each generation merely living on the top of the debris left by its predecessors. And now, as excavations have removed layer after layer, more and more primitive types of man are revealed. Just so, in disease and in dreams this control of the higher layers is lessened and the older, more primitive methods of thought reassert themselves. One can see, on this view, how natural it is for the sick person to revert to the primitive belief in magic.

Rivers did not accept Freud's conception of a censor- ship, but regarded the fantastic and symbolic forms in which hysteria and dreams manifest themselves as a regression to a lower level which was natural to the infantile stages of human development, individual or collective. He considered that a mental event could be relegated to the unconscious either by a conscious act of volition, in which case it could be recalled into consciousness, or by an "unwitting" suppression. This latter he regarded as a normal event in development and pointed out that it would be very inconvenient to the butterfly if it did not completely suppress the motor responses which had been of service to it when it was a caterpillar. Thus we reach the higher levels of our nervous system on the stepping-stones not only of our dead selves, but of our long dead ancestors.

If an animal is activated for fight or flight through the sympathetic, it may be asked how is one to account for the parasympathetic effects that are seen in overwhelming pain or fear—collapse, syncope, and loss of sphincter control? Rivers pointed out that a lowly organism has another method of defence—immobility—which takes the form in some animals of "shamming dead". Many animals, although able to perceive a moving object readily, seem to have little appreciation of a stationary one, so that immobility may prevent detection. These two methods of reaction—immobility and preparation for fight or flight—admit of no compromise. One or the other may be effective ; to attempt to combine the two would be fatal. The "all or none" principle is exemplified ; either complete immobility through the parasympathetic or violent action through the sympathetic. Thus the confusion is avoided which would inevitably result from simultaneous response of both divisions. If one comes into action the opposing group is inhibited.

But it was really not until the War that Rivers found himself and discovered his remarkable aptitude for treating the psychoneuroses. I think it was because he had had to heal himself that he could heal others. Anyhow his whole personality expanded as he grew to realize what was his true mission in life. Myers said : " He became another and a far happier man. Diffidence gave place to confidence, reticence to outspokenness, a somewhat laboured literary style to one remarkable for its ease and charm." Rivers himself said that after this war work " which brought me into contact with the real problems of life. . . . I felt that it was impossible for me to return to my life of detachment ".

Of his effect upon his patients Siegfried Sassoon has drawn a vivid picture. " Rivers never seemed elderly ; though there were more than twenty years between us, he talked as if I were his mental equal, which was very far from being the case. . . . All that matters is my remembrance of that great and good man who gave me his friendship and guidance. I can visualize him, sitting at his table in the late summer twilight, with his spectacles pushed up on his forehead and his hands clasped in front of one knee ; always communicating his integrity of mind ; never revealing that he was weary, as he must often have been after days of exceptionally tiring work on those war neuroses which demanded such an exercise of sympathy and detachment combined. . . .Quiet and alert, purposeful and unhesitating, he seemed to empty the room of everything that had needed exorcizing."

Cambridge just after the War was a strange place. Many returned thither after some years at the front and mingled with those fresh from school. There was a clash of temperaments and years. Would the old traditions re-establish themselves or should we of the pre-War generation find ourselves strangers within the walls of our own Alma Mater ? I have said before that Cambridge is adept at putting new wine into old bottles— and so it proved again. Amid changes the essentials remained. In that process Rivers played his part. His rooms were often filled with men of widely different points of view who, however, agreed in this—that here was a man who could help them and who sincerely wished to do so. His brief incursion into politics I regretted as a distraction from the work for which he was best fitted. And then in 1922, just when his influence was at its height, he died. There were enthusiastic psycho-therapists before Rivers, but the orthodox profession were inclined to regard them as cranks. But Rivers's position as an academic scientist was unassailable and his adhesion to this new branch of medicine commanded respect for it. For he was known to be " a very wise man ".

It would, I think, be fair to say that the art of medicine is the application of scientific knowledge to the relief of the individual. That there are these two aspects, and that neither is sufficient alone, must be kept in the forefront of our minds. The ultimate aim of all our training is the prevention and relief of suffering. Medicine as a pure science can never be as satisfactory as other pure sciences where the problem to be investigated can be rigidly limited and experiments carefully controlled. Our problems are generally too urgent to permit of this ; the patient has need to be relieved and that right quickly. The body of clinical evidence has to be built up slowly and fallacies in it may be difficult to detect. On the other hand medicine practised purely as an art, as in fact it was for centuries, mainly resolves itself into the exercise of the influence of a strong personality over an ailing one. It was when medical art began to rely for its data on scientific observation that it really started that extraordinarily rapid advance which the last century has seen, and which is going on with increasing acceleration. This, I fear, has led in some quarters to a persistent depreciation of the art, which is unfortunate. Clinical observation has provided much of the material for scientific research ; it hinted at the functions of each of the ductless glands before the physiological laboratory was aware of them, it provided evidence that contributed to our knowledge of the life history of the blood corpuscles, both red and white, and it advanced our knowledge of the functions of the nervous system, to quote a few examples. It was to a large extent the desire to relieve suffering that stimulated the scientific curiosity of anatomists, physiologists, and pathologists. But the art of medicine must remain. To employ a simile from the motor car again ; an engineer may know its structure and its running capacity intimately, but that in itself does not make him a skilled driver. For that road sense is required, and the factory is not the place to acquire it. The ideal conditions of the testing-room do not obtain amid crowded traffic.

To change the simile, recently within the space of four days I had the opportunity of hearing the same music performed by two pianists each of world-wide reputation. Each displayed admirable technique and execution, yet one seemed to reveal a much deeper meaning in the music than the other. And as I listened a parallel between medicine and music came into my mind. The novice finds the technique difficult to acquire, but having acquired it, it becomes second nature. That is his science. But there is practically no limit to the ways in which he can apply that technique. That is his art. The easier the technique becomes, the freer are his energies to find ever deeper meaning in his work, the more subtle his interpretations. In short, the more useful can he be to his patient and to the community.

Changing fashions in the art of medicine have their lighter side. Dr. Robert Hutchison has aptly called a fashion an epidemic fad, but considers that before the faddist can infect others and make his fad epidemic he must be a person of some importance. Smaller fashions die with or before their originator, larger ones seldom survive into the third generation. The path of medical progress is strewn with the wrecks of discarded fads; bottles of soured milk, piles of special food innocent of the smallest trace of purins, broken electrical apparatus, innumerable tablets confidently recommended by many, there they all lie. And which of us can lay his hand on his heart and truthfully say he never used any one of them? Already I see the shades of oblivion stealing over remedies popular in 1938, and I forbear to particularize. We must exercise our critical faculties and refuse to be stampeded. It is not easy, for the pressure from without is incessant. Never have people fussed more about their health than to-day. For many it

68

has replaced fussing about sin and their souls. The most alarmist ideas are promulgated ; we are a nation of degenerates, they scream, and we are poisoned by our daily food. Meanwhile, the average span of human life steadily increases and many deadly diseases have been scotched. Alarm is not the road to happiness or health. The diet faddist is perhaps the most vocal to-day. I cannot forbear to quote from Dr. Hutchison's wisdom again : " One swears by wholemeal bread, one by sour milk ; vegetarianism is the only road to salvation of some, others insist not only on vegetables alone, but on eating those raw. At one time the only thing that matters [is] calories ; at another time they are crazy about vitamins or about roughage. . . . The scientific truth may be put quite briefly ; eat moderately, having an ordinary mixed diet, and don't worry. . . . Likes and dislikes, however, should be listened to ; they are nature's indication of what probably agrees or disagrees. As to calories, our appetite . . . is usually a trustworthy guide in health. Leave raw vegetables, except salads, to the herbivorous animals. . . . There is no wonderful merit in wholemeal as opposed to ordinary bread. Don't scrape up your insides with much roughage as it is more likely to do harm than good. . . . Vegetarianism is harmless enough though it is apt to fill a man with wind and self-righteousness. . . . It is specially unsuitable for growing children and sedentary workers. Lastly it is well to remember that few diseases are caused or cured by diet alone, and that in particular diet has nothing to do with cancer. It is true, I believe, in the bodily as well as the spiritual sphere, that he who would save his life shall lose it."

* * * * *

In 292 B.C. there was a great plague in Rome, and in accordance with the advice of the sibylline books, ambassadors were sent to the Temple of Æsculapius at Epidaurus to bring his statue to Rome. As their vessel sailed up the Tiber, the story goes that a serpent which had lain concealed during the voyage, glided from it and landed among the reeds surrounding Tiber Island. This was hailed as an omen that Æsculapius himself had selected this spot. In consequence the form of a ship was given to the island and its poop can still be seen with the bust of Æsculapius with a serpent coiled round his sceptre. His temple was erected at this end of the island. When the modern embankment was made pits were found filled with votive offerings : arms, hands, feet, and three life-sized models of human trunks, cut open so as to expose the viscera, most of them in terra-cotta.

The medical history of Tiber Island goes even further back for it had previously been consecrated to a primitive Latin God—Faunus, who like Æsculapius conveyed his oracles by dreams.

In Christian times the Church of San Bartolomeo with its adjacent hospital replaced the temple. Ampère tells us when he visited this spot the Sacristan spoke of "the temple of Æsculapius, when Jove reigned", evidence of that lingering faith in paganism of which one is always faintly conscious of in Rome. Thus for more than two thousand years the island has been continuously dedicated to the spirit of healing.

When the White Ship went down and King Henry I never smiled again, his court became seriously minded. Rahere, a youth of lowly birth, had made himself popular at court by his witty talk, but when this change of thought occurred he determined to go to Rome with a view to entering the priesthood. There he was stricken with a fever, doubtless malaria, then so rife on the Campagna, and was nursed in the Hospital of San Bartolomeo on Tiber Island. In his delirium he had a vision of the apostle who told him to build a church and a hospital in Smithfield. He obeyed and the Church of St. Bartholomew the Great still stands, though in a mutilated form, and there the tomb of Rahere is still to be seen. His hospital has naturally been rebuilt several times, but for more than eight hundred years has continued its beneficent labours. Such is the link between the original Temple of Æsculapius at Epidaurus and St. Bartholomew's

Hospital. It always gratifies me therefore to regard my own hospital as, in a sense, the direct grandchild of the original temple of Æsculapius at Epidaurus.

The progress of medicine has ever been from the temple to the medical school. Though the statue of Æsculapius was carried from Epidaurus to Tiber Island, it was something more important that Rahere brought from Tiber Island to England; it was the spirit of Æsculapius opening the path to the medical school. Man is always too ready to mistake the symbol for the reality; the stone on which the laws are graven is apt to become more sacred than the laws themselves; but the statue of Æsculapius is unavailing if the spirit dies.

"JUST NERVES" [1]

How often one hears the diagnosis made, especially by laymen, of "just nerves", by which they mean that there is nothing the matter, or at least nothing more than can be put right by an effort of the will. No wonder the patient dreads the diagnosis of "just nerves", and so frequently says: "I should feel so ashamed, so humiliated, if it is just nerves."

"Just nerves" is not an imaginary illness, though it is an illness in that part of our nervous system in which our imagination has its home.

The line I take at the outset with such patients is to tell them that when I first saw in the dissecting-room the complicated network of nerves, I thought if the heart or the lungs can go wrong why should not this machinery go wrong also. Yet no one is ashamed of a disease of the heart or lungs. I admit this is not an accurate illustration, for "just nerves" is not a disturbance of peripheral nerve-trunks. In so far as the condition has a structural basis at all, it can only mean a disturbance of conduction at the contacts between association cells. But then I go on to ask why should a disturbance at this point be a subject for shame, since it is exactly the wealth of our associational powers which distinguishes us from the lower animals. There is no reason for being humiliated by a disorder of this essentially human attribute.

Yet even animals can develop functional nervous diseases, as Pavlov and Anrep showed by their experiments on conditioned reflexes. When the dog was unable readily to distinguish whether the given signal meant

[1] This and the two succeeding articles are based on clinical lectures delivered at St. Bartholomew's Hospital.

72

that he was or was not to receive food all his conditioned reflexes were upset and he became psychoneurotic. They concluded that it was an excessive demand for internal inhibition which provokes these disordered reflexes, and it is a similar demand which is at the root of many, if not most, functional nervous diseases in man.

Now I would state my views as to the origin of psycho-neuroses in a series of dogmatic propositions :

(1) To be happy in this world it is necessary to have a definite objective and an emotional interest.

(2) If these are lacking or are disappointed or come into severe conflict with other ideas there is an increased demand for internal inhibition, which we have already seen may excite an abnormal reaction even in animals if it becomes excessive.

(3) The higher levels of the nervous system are the more recent in the evolution of the race and in the development of the individual. In the disintegrative processes of disease, as Hughlings Jackson long ago pointed out, levels that are the latest to appear are the earliest to suffer.

(4) Therefore, when the demand for internal inhibition becomes excessive through failure of something necessary to happiness, the sufferer tends to revert to a habit of mind that belongs to an earlier stage in the evolution of the race or the development of the individual. This is a defence reaction, an attempt to adjust at a more primitive level.

In other words, the psychoneurotic always reverts to atavistic or infantile methods of thought. Among these we find a belief in magic and the omnipotence of thought, undue suggestibility, unreasoning terrors, undue dependence on the parent of the opposite sex, hostility towards the parent of the same sex, and a retreat from the responsibilities of adult life, which in extreme cases expresses itself as a longing for security and protection of intra-uterine existence.

Let me illustrate each of these by examples :

(1) *A belief in magic.*—Frazer points out that charms

may be based on the law of similarity, by which the magician infers that he can produce any effect he desires merely by imitating it, or on the law of contact, by which he infers that whatever he does to a material object will affect equally the person with whom the object was once in contact. The first may be called homœopathic or imitative magic, the second contagious magic.

These two principles are merely two different mis-applications of the association of ideas. Homœopathic magic commits the mistake of assuming that things which resemble each other are the same ; contagious magic commits the mistake of assuming that things which have once been in contact with each other are always in contact.

Such methods of thought may be appropriate to the ancient Hindoos, who treated jaundice by painting the patient a brighter yellow with turmeric, but it has no place in scientific medicine. Contagious magic is still exemplified in Suffolk where, if a man cuts himself with a scythe, he oils the scythe to prevent the wound from festering. A man came to a doctor with an inflamed hand, having run a thorn into it while he was hedging. On being told the hand was festering, he remarked : "That didn't ought to, for I greased the bush well arter I pulled it out " (Frazer).

Even apparently educated people believe in magical cures, such as those wrought by a certain notorious box which cures cancer, or a ring that cures rheumatism. And it is noteworthy that as a belief in magic preceded a belief in religion, so the psychoneurotic tends towards religions that emphasize the value of magical rites rather than a spiritual aspect.

(2) *The omnipotence of thought.*—" Nothing is good or ill, but thinking makes it so." The savage believes that he can have many things his own way by merely thinking they are so, the child becomes a Red Indian or a railway engine, the Christian scientist disposes of pain and sickness as a " false claim ". There are no such things because he wishes them not to be. Unfulfilled desires

may seek refuge in this omnipotence of thought. Thus an unmarried woman of 64 began to be disturbed by finding that she was the object of attention of various men whom she did not see and could not identify. Voices, however, said they wanted her. She heard the voices of the plotters arranging to take her away in a yacht. Young millionaires in motor cars kept circling round her place of residence. Here the frontiers of insanity had been definitely crossed. Less imaginative women may confine their attention to searching under the bed for a burglar. But the underlying idea is the same. Even very able men in the sorrow of a bereavement have found relief in asserting that a dead son can still smoke a cigar and drink a whisky and soda. Reality is blotted out by the strength of the wish that seeks fulfilment.

(3) *Undue suggestibility.*—All gregarious animals are suggestible, or otherwise there would be no cohesion in the herd. Man is a gregarious animal, therefore he is suggestible. And how suggestible he is advertising agents know. I recently saw it estimated that only 25 per cent of goods sold in America are really needed, the remaining 75 per cent being merely pushed on the consumer by advertisement. The advertisement columns of an American magazine are more hugely comic than any of their jokes. People lament the drink bill of England, but apparently no one was shocked, except myself, when it was triumphantly announced that our expenditure on advertisements had gone up from 100 to 150 millions. Think what it means—not only are people induced to buy what they don't want and thus waste their money ; they are also convinced of the value of many totally worthless things. During the grim days of the later part of the War almost the only smiling faces one could see were those that grinned from the hoardings, rejoicing because they had found the ideal dentifrice, the perfect cigarette, or the unbreakable sock-suspender. The obvious suggestion was to associate the ideas of purchase and happiness.

Now advertisers are practical men. They have no intention of wasting their own money, however much they intend other people to waste theirs. They know the cash value of suggestibility.

Thomas Burke has well described the clientele to which they appeal : " They are the citizens of a world of Little Pink Pamphlets and Little Daily Doses. They are the people who are shouted at, screamed at, whispered at ; commanded, cajoled, and hypnotized ; and they Eat More Fruit when they are told to, and Drink More Milk ; Get that Worth-While Feeling and they Say it with Flowers and Go to Sunny Sunport for their Holidays ; and they Keep that Schoolgirl Complexion and believe that Good Cigarettes are a Perfect Digestive. . . . And over them the guardian angel of stunt and slogan drops his crooked laughter " (*The Sun in Splendour*).

If the average man is thus suggestible, how much more suggestible is the man sick in body or in mind ! He is at the mercy of the first person he meets with a quack recipe in his pocket. I feel very strongly that it is the duty of the medical man not to suggest ill-health.

(4) *Unreasoning terrors.*—Fear is a defensive mechanism, of obvious survival value ; unreasoning fear is a perversion of this defensive mechanism, usually arising from some internal conflict or the persistence of some early painful impression. Phobias are a reversion to the night terrors of childhood or to the mentality of a savage, who walks all his days hedged in between totem and taboo. H. G. Wells reminds us that the savage is really far more neurotic than civilized man—a fact we are very apt to ignore.

Well, as Jane Harrison remarked, man has got to be afraid of something. He's no longer afraid of hell, so he has to be afraid of germs, of cancer or what you will.

As Havelock Ellis said : " When other animals cease to torture [man] he must torture himself. Having destroyed the wolf, man must become a wolf unto himself. When he has destroyed the natural causes of fear it is inevitable that he should replace them by substitutes."

Unreasoning terrors form such a large part of the sufferings of the neurotic that it will be well to consider the mechanism by which we all experience fear. When organisms were still of a lowly structure their internal life was simple and could still be carried on by chemical mechanisms. But they required an "awareness" of their environment, a capacity to avoid danger and to seek food. Thus it happened that sensitive perceptive structures were first developed on the surface of their bodies. The nervous system, therefore, started in the skin, but the nerve cells soon withdrew themselves into a more protected position. Without going into all the details of the building up of the nervous system, we find that the portion known as the sympathetic nervous system, which superintends many of the functions of organic life, retains some of the primitive features of the nervous system of lower animals. Its response is urgent, immediate, widespread and explosive. It is brought into action by pain, rage, fear, and any intense excitement. Dr. W. B. Cannon pointed out that the effects of sympathetic stimulation were all originally designed to activate the body for a struggle and to increase its power of defence. Reserves are freely spent now to produce energy just as they were formerly spent to aid the primitive animal in its struggle with its antagonists. It has been well said that the sympathetic nervous system responds in the same way to fight, fright, or flight. Dr. G. W. Crile has illustrated this by a modern instance and a modern simile : "And now, though sitting at his desk in command of the complicated machinery of civilization, man's fear is manifested in terms of his ancestral physical battle in the struggle for existence. He cannot fear intellectually, he cannot fear dispassionately ; he fears with all his organs, and the same organs are stimulated and inhibited as if it were a physical battle with teeth and claws. . . . Nature has the one means of response to fear and, whatever its cause, the response

77

is always the same, always physical. . . . Under modern conditions of life neither fight nor flight is *de rigueur*. The individual under the stimulation of fear may be likened to an automobile with the clutch thrown out, but whose engine is racing at full speed. The gasoline is being consumed, the machinery is being worn out, but the machine as a whole does not move, though the power of its engine may cause it to tremble." Professor William McDougall gives us another reason for this similarity of response of the sympathetic nervous system to different emotions when he points out how all the instinctive impulses, when met with opposition, give rise to or are complicated by the combative instinct which is directed against the source of opposition. The dog threatened with the loss of the bone he is eating, the conflict of the males for the possession of a mate, the maternal instinct converted into anger of combat against an attempt to injure her young are examples which will occur to the mind at once. There is, indeed, as Cannon says, obvious reason why the visceral changes in fear and rage should not be different but why they should be so alike : for these emotions are both accompanied by organic preparations for action.

We are certainly justified in stating that a state of continued fear, whether recognized or not as such by the sufferer, is capable of producing the symptoms of which they so generally complain. Moreover, I believe that the great majority of such manifestations are of that order.

" Emotion moves us, hence the name," said Sherrington. It would perhaps be more accurate to say that it is designed to move us. When under conditions of modern life, emotion is dissociated from the movement it should evoke under more primitive conditions, the sympathetic disturbance may continue. The mobilized army which is not allowed to fight the enemy becomes a danger to its own country. The animal that is restrained from fight or flight suffers an increased fear.

We are now in a position to understand two things. The first is why the neurotic should refer so many of his

78

symptoms to disorders in various organs, for we see that the emotional disturbance leads to preparation in them for intense activity, and the disturbances will persist because that activity has not taken place and, as it were, cleared them off. The second is why he should suffer from such terrors and phobias. Fear is really a perversion of a defensive mechanism of great antiquity and is specially intense when there is interference with any form of reaction to danger. We must not regard the response of an animal to danger as having the full emotional strength of what we mean by fear. To do so would be to fall into the common error of interpreting the activities of the simpler animals as though they were miniature human beings. The much scantier associative mechanisms in the nervous system of lower animals precludes such an idea. The late A. C. Benson said : " It is strange to note the perpetual instinctive consciousness of danger which besets birds in the open ; they must live in a tension of nervous watchfulness which would depress a human being into melancholia. . . . Do we realize what it must be to live, as even sheltered birds do, in a quiet garden, with the fear of an attack and death hanging over them from morn to night ? " The best answer to this anthropomorphic view is that the behaviour of birds gives no suggestion of their being depressed into melancholia. Doubtless, when the appropriate motor response is prevented, the lower animal feels both pain and fear, but that all its sensations and emotions are thus coloured is most improbable, when we consider the much simpler structure of its nervous system.

It might be argued, on the other hand, that, as sensations of fear arise at once when the controlling mechanism is in abeyance, as in night terrors or in states of exhaustion, this might suggest that fear must be a primitive emotion of great strength and universally present in lower forms of life. But I would urge that such fears belong to the phase when the nervous system has reached a sufficiently high stage of development to feel them, but not a sufficiently high one to control them.

79

Fear is not a necessary accompaniment of consciousness, it is a product of self-consciousness.

The behaviour of savages supports this view. Fear, whether of evil spirits, of magic, of the dark, panic fear dominated primitive man and, whenever our resistance is lowered by disease, by shock, or by psychic conflict, we betray our ancestry. That strange, primitive being which lurks in the unconscious mind of us all, peeps out. Elaboration of ceremonial and ritual is the first step taken by primitive man to counteract this ; all religions pass through the " God-fearing " stage. Then with the higher development of the mind, and the recognition of the reality principle, comes release from such obsessions of fear.

But under certain conditions this higher control fails and phobias develop. The alertness in the presence of danger that is normal and necessary to an animal is apt to be translated into unreasoning fear in man.

We must now go a stage further and inquire why the cause of the phobia is so generally unrecognized by the sufferer. It has been well said that life is a compromise between our instincts and our conventions. For the neurotic, life is a conflict between them. The energy generated by the instincts soon finds itself opposed by conditions of the environment—the irresistible force and the immovable obstacle again. Either this energy has to be sublimated, i.e. diverted into other and higher channels compatible with social conditions, or it has to be repressed. If repression fails the energy rises by devious routes into consciousness and produces painful conflicts. The memories and the pain arising from them become associated like conditioned reflexes.

I have already mentioned " conditioned reflexes ". May I recall what is meant by that term ; an animal has a secretion of saliva when it is given or shown food. If a bell is sounded every time the food is given, it soon happens that the sound of the bell will cause secretion, even when there is no food. Many similar examples could be quoted. The behaviour of shell-shocked soldiers has been compared to these conditioned reflexes. Thus in some cases the noise of a tin can recall the warning signal of a gas attack, and the screech of the overhead wire of a tram recalled the sound of a shell coming over. They responded to these sounds as they did in the War, though they had forgotten why they did so. Just as the animal may come to secrete saliva when the bell is sounded although no food is there, so the soldiers may have a paroxysm of fear when the warning sound is given although no danger exists. Similar associations can also be traced in the neuroses of civilian life. On conditioned reflexes quite complicated associations may be built up, and in all probability they form the foundation of much of our psychic life. When a memory is called into consciousness the emotion associated with the original incident may be revived. But the curious part of it is that the emotion may be evoked more rapidly than the memory. When the memory is a painful one the emotion may play the part of a defence reaction by producing a disturbance which distracts attention from the cause. The danger signal is raised and the response to it occurs without the memory becoming a conscious one. Now the patient's lack of knowledge of the mechanism concerned allows a state of anxiety to arise. The relationship of cause and effect is not comprehended. Mystery produces fear. This emotional response may be aroused more quickly than the memory, even when it is a pleasant one. One day I was walking through Pump Court in the Temple in London, when suddenly I felt extraordinarily happy. Then I recognized that the feeling of happiness was associated with the noise of a can being filled at a stand pipe. Then I knew that it recalled the noise my college servant made filling the water-can for the bath that awakened me when an undergraduate at Cambridge, when to awaken was to anticipate another delightful day. Here there was no need for the memory to be repressed, and it was not ; but there was a perceptible interval of time between the emotion and the memory. When the memory is repressed because it is painful, the apparent causelessness of the emotion in itself excites alarm, and what ultimate form of expression that alarm takes will depend on many factors in the individual and the environment.

With continued repression the impulses arising from the unconscious attempt to reach the surface by more and more devious routes. As their association with the painful memory becomes dimly recognized the area of repressed ideas spreads until only in a distorted form widely removed from the original cause do they attain a conscious level. Thus a lady who had undergone a painful experience in York not only refused to go to York again, which is comprehensible, but she would become agitated at the sight of a train whose destination was labelled York. She would cross out the name York in a time-table. All this, of course, is clearly connected with the fact that the idea of going to York was disagreeable to her. But later on she displayed an aversion to York ham, Yorkshire pudding, and Yorkshire relish, all of which she had previously liked. The attempt to obliterate painful memories spread to everything connected with the name of York. This shows how an attack of " nerves " may be excited by something which seems curiously remote from the original cause.

(5) *Psychoneurotic reactions between parent and child.*— There is no more disastrous fallacy in conventional thought than that the relationship between parent and child is naturally easy and simple. It is far better to realize that difficulties inevitably arise, difficulties which call for consideration and courage on both sides. Parental love is instinctive and possessive, and the child, as he or she grows up, may find one of two difficulties—either a tendency to excessive dependence as in the days of infancy, or a resistance on the parent's part to the children establishing their own individuality. " A child rightly brought up will be like a willow branch which, broken off and touching the ground, at once takes root. Bring up your children so that they will root easily in their own soil, and not for ever be grafted into your old trunk and boughs " (Henry Ward Beecher). Too often the parent

expects the child to be a replica, an extension of his own ego—which, considering the care Nature has taken to kaleidoscope the chromosomes, is as impossible as it is undesirable in the interests of the race. Undue dependence is more likely between the parent and child of opposite sex, antagonism between those of the same sex. For this reason alone a real sex war is impossible.

Anorexia nervosa, a psychoneurosis in girls after puberty, accompanied by amenorrhœa and self-starvation is, in my experience, invariably associated with a hostility towards the mother. But this hostility may show itself much earlier, and I recently came across a case of a female child of two who displayed tragic misery in the presence of her mother. She was unwilling to take food, and such as she did take disagreed with her. Yet with her grandmother she was quite happy, ate well and put on weight rapidly. I have never come across another instance so early in life as this.

A doctor friend of mine had a small boy of 7 who displayed anger whenever his father kissed his mother, and would then often strike his father. They thought it amusing, and actually " showed off " this accomplishment of his to me. His father was quite surprised when I warned him of the trouble they were preparing for the future.

I should like to refer to two cases of psychoneuroses which developed in successful professional men in their conflict to detach themselves from the overwhelming influence of the mother.

One of these, a man now 42, has consulted me at intervals for over ten years. After two great shocks during the war he developed extraordinary vasomotor disturbances, which have continued at intervals ever since. Various endocrine symptoms followed, which led some physicians he saw to label him as hypopituitarism at one time, hypoadrenalism at another, and so on. He consulted an eminent German physician who said that there was no disease of any gland, but a loss of balance between them, so that sometimes one and sometimes another gland appeared to be affected. My contention was that the disturbed balance and the vasomotor troubles must be due to some common factor, and that the only common factor I could suggest was the sympathetic nervous system. And, further, that though shock could affect the sympathetic nervous system, the effect could not be so prolonged unless there was some continuing psychological cause. This suggestion always seemed to annoy him. He maintained that there must be a physical cause which I could not find out. He went on to say that he was surprised that I, with a presumably scientific training, should say such a thing. Mind and body were quite distinct and could not influence one another. I could only retort that for a presumably intelligent man to say such a thing showed that he had some reason for denying their obvious interactions. Moreover, I thought to myself, a man does not keep coming for ten years and paying me fees for telling him something he really thinks nonsense. Well, a few weeks ago he suddenly blurted out the secret he had so carefully denied the existence of—his mother, now aged 70, has always tried to drive a wedge in between his wife and himself. He had told me that he dated his nervous troubles from his marriage, which had led me to a natural but evidently erroneous conclusion. His wife and he were much attached to each other and his mother's attitude was disastrous to his health. If he could detach himself from maternal influence—for this is a case where compromise is impossible—the conflict would be over. But he can't make up his mind to this. However, when his mother objected to his going to the seaside this summer with his wife and children and said he ought to stay with her, I urged him to go. He went, and his health improved until he came under her influence again. I need hardly add that his mother is convinced that I do not understand his case.

The second case is one of a man of about the same age, whose mother died a year and a half ago ; yet he cannot free himself from her dominating influence.

During the War he attempted to do so and there was a tremendous scene when he joined up. Wires were pulled and he found himself transferred to a "cushy job". This produced an internal conflict because, as he said : "He was not any more anxious to be killed than anyone else." He had a phobia about going for railway journeys because in early life she had instilled in him a fear of meeting hostile strangers under these conditions, with the object of keeping him with her. He had a phobia about catching cold, because at the slightest sign of a cold she had put him to bed for two or three days. He asked if he could carry on his work if he did get an ordinary cold. I replied: "Yes ; it is better for you to be free than safe."

Note that both these patients were highly successful professional men. Psychoneuroses are not confined to incompetent fools.

(6) *Retreat from life.*—A woman in the thirties, on her father's death, bought a property in the country. Here she lives with her mother, a big dog, and as few servants as possible. Within a ring fence she made the house and grounds as beautiful as she could. She has good taste, and every detail has been thought out with meticulous care. She wishes for no visitors, and here, secluded from the world, she intended to be completely happy. But Nature took her revenge for this retreat from life, and she has been afflicted with one psychoneurosis after another. And she will continue to be as long as she persists in her present attitude ; no ring fence will shut out psychoneuroses. For, as Maurice Nicoll says : "The psyche is not designed to be stationary, and if we seek to be static and to cling to outlived values in ourselves we must inevitably suffer, because we shall be at war with a principle *in* ourselves, not outside ourselves, although we may see it only so." And he claims that in human psychology is embodied a dynamic principle, the denial of which must produce psychological unhappiness.

Women are essentially more static than men. They

85

may change their fashions more readily, but they cling to their earlier views more than men. For this reason they must be more subject to psychoneuroses than men. Hence, too, their amazing self-pity in a world which will keep changing.

But men and woman alike who retreat from life will suffer and they will degenerate. Complete withdrawal means complete dementia.

A psychoneurosis may also have its origin in some strong instinctive impulse which is repressed as being inconsistent with the conscious standards of the individual. To me it seemed extraordinary that the censor who at first vetoed a beautiful play like *Young Woodley* permitted the production of a homosexual sadistic horror like *The Man with Red Hair*. But perhaps he did not realize what it meant ; that would be quite in accordance with the traditions of an office which censored serious artists like Ibsen and Bernard Shaw. I am sure from clinical experience that the state of mind which Sir Hugh Walpole describes in that play lies at the root of a good many psychoneuroses, although usually the real cause is unknown to the sufferer. I had a case in which the patient had a phobia of the sight of blood, leading to fainting attacks in specially unpleasant circumstances. This was traced to a repressed cruelty lust, and the gradual bringing of this to the patient's knowledge was followed by relief of his symptoms.

Now I want strongly to insist that it is not the frankly cruel man or woman (and these cases are at least as common in what is grotesquely termed the " gentler sex ") who suffer from psychoneuroses as a result. It is the better type, where the cruel, sadistic trend is at war with the rest of the personality, who suffer in this way. I was recently much struck by a paragraph in an essay by Aldous Huxley on a picture by Brueghel of the Crucifixion in which the scene is represented as one of frank enjoyment for the spectators. He goes on to say : " At Tyburn one could get an excellent seat in a private box for half a crown ; with the ticket in one's pocket one could follow the cart all the way from the prison, arrive with the criminal and yet have a perfect view of the performance. In these later days, when cranky humanitarianism has so far triumphed that hangings take place in private and Mrs. Thompson's screams are not even allowed to be recorded on the radio, we have to be content with reading about executions, not with seeing them. The impresarios who sold seats at Tyburn have been replaced by titled newspaper proprietors who sell juicy descriptions of Tyburn to a prodigiously much larger public."

" That eager, tremulous, lascivious interest in blood and beastliness which in these more civilized days we can only satisfy at one remove from reality in the pages of our newspapers, was franklier indulged in Brueghel's day ; the naïve, ingenuous brute in man was less sophisticated, was given longer rope, and joyously barks and wags its tail round the appointed victim."

Allowing for Aldous Huxley's taste for invective, I think this puts the case powerfully and well. Man has not found it easy to " let the ape and tiger die " within him. It is a commonplace of embryology that all life has to repeat in brief and with modifications the history of the race. A strain of cruelty seems normal in the healthy child at a certain age, restrained though it is by the pressure of social convention. But if it persists, one of two things happens : either the individual remains a brute, or he finds a war in his members going on— when he would do good, evil is present with him. He attempts to push the hideous thing out of his consciousness, and unfortunately often only succeeds in pushing it down to the unconscious level, where it still remains a source of conflict. Whether Nature abhors a vacuum or not, it is certainly true that the chamber will not remain swept and garnished ; a positive evil cannot be exorcized by a mere negative—it must be replaced by something equally positive.

But now I come to a very mysterious part of these

cases ; when the cruelty trend is found to be only displayed by the patient towards an individual or a representative of a class, you may be pretty certain he is searching for a scapegoat. Frankly, I mean in so many words that he is venting on someone else the discomfort and dissatisfaction he feels for something wrong in himself. How utterly illogical, you may say. But is not the search for a scapegoat an extraordinarily deeply rooted instinct in human nature ?

Plenty of illustrations must spring to mind of all. As a race evolves, its ideas of a scapegoat become less crude and less cruel. Human sacrifice is replaced by animal sacrifice and then by symbolic substitutes for a sacrifice at all. But the psychoneurotic, with his atavistic trends, finds himself desiring, even against his better judgment, the cruder method, and you have got to find out what is the obsession from which he is trying to find release by seeking a scapegoat.

I want to make a plea for the psychoneurotic. Even in medical circles there is still too much of a tendency to despise him. I have been trying to show that he is a man struggling to adapt himself to evolutionary requirements. If he were not struggling he would not suffer—he, like the crowd at Tyburn, would be content to remain adapted to a lower level. But you may ask, why is he struggling if he does not know what is the matter with him, and how can explanation of the facts help him ?

These are the points on which Freud has thrown so much light. I may say at once that while regarding Freud as one of the most original thinkers of our time, I by no means accept his doctrine entire. I reserve the right of private judgment, and consider that he bases his views on too narrow a conception. Now this is exactly what the convinced Freudian will not allow you to do. It is extraordinary to see this development of a new orthodoxy, from which you must not dissent if you are to be saved. The Freudian creed is of the straightest. There is one God, the subconscious, and Freud is his prophet. There are the sacred books, which you must accept as literally true. You must not inquire, "What do I find? What is my own experience," or you will be told, "This fellow does not know what Freud said on the subject." Finally we have the heresy hunt, and Adler and Jung must be solemnly excommunicated with bell, book, and candle. Now this is a preposterous attitude to adopt on any scientific subject. Where should we be in physics if we had made Newton's Laws of Motion or Dalton's Atomic Theory into an Athanasian creed? Strange that men, having emancipated themselves from one orthodoxy, should straightway desire to shackle themselves in another. Evidently there is a good deal of the old Adam even in the mental processes of Freudians. But particularly is this attitude absurd when applied to such unexplored territory as the subconscious mind. To claim that the first prospector of it should discover the truth, the whole truth, and nothing but the truth is to demand too much of human credulity. Nevertheless, I am convinced that Freud's main conception as to the way in which the subconscious behaves is right. And I am convinced for the best of reasons—that in practice it works. It helps one to discover the cause of the patient's trouble.

I must remind you that none of these patients come or are sent to me because they are thought to be suffering from a psychoneurosis. If that were so they would go elsewhere—to recognized psychotherapists. They come to me in the belief that they are suffering from some organic or, at least, some tangible disease, and on investigation I find reason to believe that they are not. Almost invariably the outward and visible evidence of their condition is some cardiac or vasomotor symptom— syncopal attacks, cold, white or cyanotic extremities, sweats, respiratory distress, sudden darting pains in the head or elsewhere, paræsthesiæ, exhaustion, and collapse. With these invariably goes an overmastering sense of fear. The patient thinks the fear is the result of the distressing symptom, whereas the symptom is really the consequence of fear.

Note particularly that the reaction is uncomprehended. The fact that the body acts in this incomprehensible way materially increases the fear aroused. It is no use for the patient to be told to fight against it, for the will has not control over the unknown. The cause of the conflict must be brought up into consciousness before the will can have any power over it. It may well be that in attempting to do this we shall meet with great resistance. It is unusual to meet with a patient who accepts the situation frankly. It is more usual for them to shy as the method of free association brings them nearer to the painful spot. They will say, " I don't know why I said that," or " That's nothing to do with it," or they will pass into mulish silence. When the painful memory is actually awakened there will probably be an emotional outburst. This, according to one school, is an important factor in treatment—abreaction as it is called. I am not so convinced of this as I am that it is an important indication that the real source of the trouble has been detected.

When the cause has been found the further treatment of the case may still present difficulties. Freud lays great stress on what he calls positive transference, which really amounts to an emotional dependence on the medical man. That in all cases of illness, whether mental or physical, a bond of sympathy between doctor and patient is an important thing is, of course, well recognized—we can do little good where we are not trusted. It is the particular merit of the English system of clinical training that from the very first the student is given the opportunity of coming into personal contact with the patients and thereby of acquiring this important kind of experience and skill. But positive transference may become a danger, or at least a hindrance, if carried too far—the patient becomes too dependent on the doctor when we want him to stand on his own feet. I think, therefore, that quite early in the treatment attempts should be made to find an outlet for the energy which is released on relieving the internal friction and it is astonishing how much energy can be wasted over merely maintaining an internal inhibition—witness the exhaustion which is so common a symptom in such cases. This energy must be sublimated into some positive occupation in which the patient's emotional interest is actively aroused.

The psychoneurosis may express itself at one or more of the three levels of the nervous system :

(1) *At the psychical level* by phobias, obsessions, and compulsion neuroses.

(2) *At the sensori-motor level* by paralyses, tremors, tics, and anæsthesias.

(3) *At the vegetative level*, though here a toxic factor may often determine the form the symptoms take, such as vasomotor disturbances, palpitation, hyper-thyroidism, asthma, atonic dilatation of the stomach, glycosuria.

In determining whether a patient's condition is due to a psychoneurosis, great attention must be paid to taking the history. It will soon appear that the symptoms are inconsistent with any known organic disease. This must be followed by a routine physical examination, paying careful attention to all points where the patient complains of symptoms. If this is omitted he will not believe that you have excluded organic disease. While the patient is still lying quietly on the examining couch, inquire into ordinary sources of worry and anxiety. If the cause is at a conscious level it will probably come out with sympathetic handling. Remember that it is easier to say things behind your back than to your face, and give opportunities for this. If the cause is not at a conscious level, other methods, such as that of free association and analysis of dreams, may help to throw light on it. But it is not possible here to discuss the details of all this. It is most important never to show surprise and particularly no disgust. It is surprising how frequently without formal psycho-analysis it is possible to help the patient by bringing the repressed idea into conscious-ness. For then the will can bring it into relation with its rational self, whereas the will cannot control what it does not know. " Fighting " a phobia, the cause of which is unknown, appears merely to strengthen its hold, whereas an explanation of its cause may lead to its disappearance.

I am convinced that more and more we shall have to realize and to treat the psychological aspects of disease. This conviction has simply been forced upon me by the experiences of practice. In my student days little attention was paid to functional nervous disease. I have myself heard the patient told, " The cure rests mainly with yourself." True in a sense, but the patient has to be shown the way. The late Dr. Crookshank humorously expressed the orthodox view thus : " Organic is what we say we cure, but don't ; while functional disease is what the quacks cure and we wish that we could." I believe that quite as many people are ill because they are unhappy as are unhappy because they are ill.

This method of approach to your work will make it infinitely more interesting. It will add to the sense of responsibility with which you enter the patient's house, for you will become a trusted confidant. It is in consequence of these developments that the doctor is becoming the recipient of confidences rather than the clergyman, who is suspected of having a standardized remedy for all psychical ills. The doctor of the future will have to come doubly armed—with material aids for material troubles, and with psychotherapy for distresses of the spirit.

NEW PAINS FOR OLD

The two things which bring a patient to a doctor are fear and pain. These may co-exist in very varying degree. I have already said that the unknown is a very potent factor in exciting fear. It is extraordinary to see how a definite diagnosis, even if not an entirely favourable one, may relieve the patient's mind. Pain, even severe pain, may not be accompanied by fear if the cause be known. But under certain conditions pain may be accompanied by a sense of impending dissolution, which excites the most distressing fears, the " angor animi " of the ancient writers, " that sense of ruin that is worse than pain," a condition not simply confined to dangerous diseases.

The origin of fear has already been briefly discussed. What are the characteristic features, physiologically speaking, of pain ?   Other sensations are conveyed through touch corpuscles of varying structure and complexity.   Naked nerve endings can apparently only convey one kind of sensation—that of pain—*vide* those on the surface of the eyeball. Any nerve ending, clothed or naked, if adequately stimulated, can flare up into urgent messages of pain.   But the end organ allows of discrimination and it can register an impression too slight to cause pain.   Thus the retina can convey the sensation of a dim light, while a blinding light may cause actual pain. The sensation of pain is not so easily elicited, but once it is aroused it is explosive in character and prolonged. To illustrate this from a familiar fact. At the right temperature water will give merely a pleasant sensation of warmth, but if you put your hand in water that is just too hot the painful sensation comes perceptibly later than that of warmth. You may be able to bear the immersion of the hand, but if you increase the stimulated area by plunging in the whole arm, the number of painful impressions will mount up unbearably. Moreover the pain will persist after you have withdrawn your arm because, as Sir Thomas Lewis has shown, a chemical substance, exciting pain, has been set free. As we know, these painful sensations pass by their own special tract in the spinal cord, and at a special rate. They arrive in the brain at the thalamus which is the older, more primitive, receptive structure than the sensory cortex. It is the latter which enables attention to be concentrated on any part of the body that is stimulated. The sensations received there are also brought into relation with other sensory processes, past and present. The sensory cortex, in fact, contributes towards a control over feelings and has the power within limits to decide how to act. Thus the same painful message may result in the recipient launching out a violent blow against the offender, or the cortex, recognizing that the pain is due to the knife of the surgeon, cruel only to be kind, inhibits movement of the part attacked, and diverts its energy into a loud yell. Or the attention of the cortex may be diverted, so that the painful stimulus is not felt, and a man is unaware of a wound received in the excitement of battle. Owing to such cortical control the hysterical patient may experience nothing from the prick of a pin.

Ordinary sensations, then, have a low threshold, they enter the nervous system easily, and as Adrian has shown, travel rapidly ; they are dealt with by the brain according to its needs and moods ; sensations of pain have a higher threshold, not gaining admission so easily nor travelling so fast, but once admitted may give rise to a positive explosion of nervous activity.

That pain, like fear, is a defensive mechanism is obvious. Indeed it is one of the highest value. I remember reading a tale when I was a child of a woodcutter who was promised by a fairy godmother that one wish should be fulfilled. Smarting from a recent wound from his axe, he wished that he should not feel pain. In a short time he had cut and burnt himself so severely that he died. I always imagine that this story must have been based on a case of syringomyelia. Years ago a philosophic surgeon, James Hilton, wrote a medical classic entitled *Rest and Pain*, stressing the value of pain as ensuring rest. The late Sir James Mackenzie also pointed out the value of cardiac pain in preventing over-exertion for a damaged heart. But unfortunately pain, as I have already said, may persist after its value as a warning signal is past. Pain then becomes a portent of a distressing kind. Both fear and pain present difficulties to the doctor which are all the greater because there is no objective standard by which to measure them. Dilatation of the pupil, acceleration of the pulse, and even the galvanopsychic reflex are not really adequate to do so. The personal factor is enormous. Lombroso maintained that habitual criminals, particularly those who are addicted to crimes of great violence and brutality, have a marked degree of indifference to pain in themselves. In this matter extremes meet, for highly sensitive mystics and martyrs may in their state of spiritual exaltation show a similar indifference to pain. H. G. Wells in *The Research Magnificent* has a pertinent observation on this point. He makes one of his characters remark : " We exaggerate the range of pain as if it were limitless. We think . . . that it passes into agony and so beyond endurance to destruction. It probably does nothing of the kind. . . . The recorded behaviour of martyrs or the self-torture of Hindoo ascetics, or the defiance of Red Indian prisoners . . . are they really horrible at all ? It is possible that these charred and slashed and splintered persons, these Indians hanging from hooks, have had glimpses through great windows that were worth the price they paid for them ? "

Here we touch the fringe of a psychological mystery. It may be that to-day we tend to undervalue the spiritual exaltation that may accompany pain, as much as it seems to us to have been over valued in the past. A distinguished colleague of mine, Professor C. E. Raven, has put on record a terribly poignant account of his sufferings from a painful accident, but he bears witness to the extraordinary exaltation which accompanied it. But I think he is of the stuff of which martyrs were made, and I doubt whether to-day many of us would submit to torture over theological differences, as many did in the past with apparent gladness. It may well be that analgesics and anæsthetics have, by abolishing so much pain, made us more sensitive to what remains. To most of us the sufferings endured in the past seem frankly intolerable. But I note a tendency of some modern novelists, such as Cowper Powys, to dwell on the psychological concomitants of pain with undisguised gusto. I must say I do not like that attitude ; the frontiers of sadism are soon crossed.

For despite all that poets and moralists have written, and all that martyrs and mystics have endured, pain appears to the medical man to be an evil. He sees many more characters deteriorated than elevated by prolonged pain. I have read with deep sympathy the graphic and courageous account by a surgical friend of his unbearable sufferings from the agonies of thrombarteritis obliterans, but I note that it was when the pain was relieved by amputation that he was able to acquire a gracious and philosophical calm. Indeed, Schopenhauer rated the cessation of pain as one of the few positive pleasures in this world. It may well be that it is just because I have experienced singularly little pain in my life that I regard it as an evil. But it is one of the curious facts about pain that it is usually speedily forgotten, which hardly argues that it is a good thing. Anyhow we doctors are called upon to relieve it, and relieve it we must if we can. It is not for us of all people to argue as to its possible benefits.

And here we are up against another difficulty. Hippocrates, the father of medicine, said: " Of simultaneous pain in two places, the lesser is obliterated by the greater." Which is greater, physical or mental pain ? Few would doubt that the latter is worse. Certainly

96

medical men are constantly seeing instances where patients seek a physical pain as the relief to mental pain. For the former can be talked about and will excite sympathy ; the latter they prefer to bury in their own bosoms. And then comes the magician, offering new lamps for old, new pains for old, and pains that can be talked about. In our work we must be constantly on the watch for these substitute pains and search for the underlying mental or emotional cause. By concentrating sufficient attention on any part of our anatomy we can develop a pain there, and it is all the easier to have that pain if at the same time the emotional sympathetic nervous system is keyed up. I imagine that the stigmata of saints, if not self-produced, were self-induced in some such way.

To take a simple instance in the first place. A woman who has brought up several children has had all her energies fully absorbed for a number of years. Child-bearing absorbs much that would otherwise go in other directions. Two able women have independently testified to me as to the great difficulty they experienced in sustained directed thinking when they were pregnant. In course of time the family grows up and she finds herself without any invested capital of mental interests. Then she has an illness ; the family comes rushing back to the bedside ; once again the household revolves about her. The lesson is learned and advantage is taken of it and she proceeds, in the illuminating phrase, to " enjoy ill-health ".

The doctor's position is difficult—if he were to divulge his opinion he would be regarded as a hard-hearted brute who doesn't know his business. Of course, gradually one other person comes to recognize the true state of affairs—the husband. But he doesn't tell, not even to the doctor, unless he is very tactfully cross-examined—and sometimes not even then. His wife may criticize him lavishly at afternoon tea-tables, but if he criticizes her at his club you may conclude he was very drunk indeed. There is a lot of quiet heroism in unsuspected places.

97   H

I am not implying that the fault is always on one side. I remember an interesting case of heroism in a woman which exactly illustrates my point. The patient was a young woman who had had an unhappy childhood ; her parents quarrelled incessantly ; her mother was drunken and vicious. She then had a happy time as a schoolmistress, for this satisfied her evidently strong maternal instincts. She married a man much older than herself chiefly from motives of pity. She had a great shock on finding that he was determined not to have children. He would not even allow her to have a dog. She began to suffer from severe abdominal pains.

I came to the conclusion that she was deliberately constipating herself because the resulting physical pains distracted her mind from mental pain. I taxed her with this, and having gained her confidence she told me the facts I have mentioned and admitted the point. She got very much better, and free from pain, but unfortunately became obsessed with the advantages of self-starvation. She became easier in mind but much weaker in body. I saw her again after an interval of two years and was shocked by the change in her, but she was now quite bright and apparently happy. Asceticism had provided her with a way of escape from mental woes. She adopted the Salisbury treatment and took the most meticulous care in cleansing the meat from every trace of fat or connective tissue. Her small meal required about two hours to prepare and even longer to eat ! I strongly suspect these self-starvers and purifiers to be haunted by an obsession of sin, though in this case it may have been prompted by a desire for vicarious sacrifice.

These new self-inflicted pains may be a protective mechanism, as in the case of a girl in the early twenties who took to her bed for a couple of years on account of abdominal pains for which no one could find a cause, and which she would not have investigated by modern methods. Some time after, her father died and left her sufficient money to be independent. She rose from her bed, quarrelled with her mother, and ran away with the married chauffeur, who beats her, but her former pains have vanished.

Another example of protective pains is the following. A young married woman was sent to see me because of a story of extraordinary pains in all sorts of places. Like many another she was the subject of cancerphobia. She was anxious to go into a nursing home for observation and treatment but discharged herself within twenty-four hours, leaving an address to which I could send a note of fees, which, needless to say, I never received. The mechanism here was fairly obvious ; her husband had obtained a post in India, and she hated the life there. She complained of her health so much that at last, in sheer desperation he told her to come home and not to return until she was cured. As she does not want to return there is very little probability of her being cured. The more doctors she consults the more she can impress her husband with her efforts to be cured, and the fewer of those doctors she pays the longer this process can last.

Another case of cancerphobia in a patient of a higher level of intelligence was in a man of about fifty, with nervous dyspepsia. He had lost his wife, to whom he was devoted, from cerebral hæmorrhage after an air raid. He was left with four small children, and a widow with one child of her own offered to look after them if he would marry her. He did so and life became almost impossible. He had to fight for his children's rights against the favouritism she extended to her child. During the food rationing in the later stages of the War he found this child was being surreptitiously fed at the expense of his. He had no escape for his work was done at home—he had no mitigation by getting away to business for the greater part of the day. He had an invalid mother dependent on him, and he had to go on working whether he felt ill or not. Gradually he came to think that only death could bring him any relief, and then the thought came—but it might be death by cancer ; that would be a horrible way out. And so the phobia grew and his misery increased.

Indecision may be an important factor in producing

substitute pains, as in a girl of 21 who was engaged to be married. As she was an only child a conflict arose in her mind between a disinclination to leave the security of home life and a natural impulse to assume more adult responsibilities. This concentrated her mind very much upon her own health, because unsatisfactory health enabled her to hold the balance between these two factors in the conflict. I told her and her doctor that I believed that as long as she remained in this state of indecision her health would suffer and I urged that she should go ahead with her arrangements to get married. She did so and got quite well. That was nearly two years ago—but recently she has relapsed, again on account of indecision. Her husband wants a child, and she is fearful of taking on such a responsibility. So again bad health is invoked, and again I have urged her to decide in favour of completing her adult existence.

Recently I saw a girl whose health had seriously failed ; no objective cause could be found for this beyond a slight swelling of the thyroid, without any real evidence of hyperthyroidism. On inquiry I found that she had been teaching in a school where her cousin was the wife of the headmaster. She liked the life ; threw herself into it with enthusiasm, and gave out a lot of energy. She had made good, and then her cousin's attitude towards her changed—no rival was to be permitted near the throne —and she was subjected to a series of pinpricks. While having to do the social things that might be looked for in a relation, at other times she was kept rigidly at arm's length as a member of the staff. She felt this very much, and it was a disillusionment to her enthusiastic nature to find herself punished for her successful devotion to her work. Her thyroid began to swell at this time. It is rather significant that her thyroid had been noted to swell on a former occasion, when she had some little disagreement with her father about the work she was to undertake. There had also been somewhat of a disappointment because one of the under-masters became engaged to someone else. Her experience of the outside world after the protection of home life had been too hard and disillusioning ; it had thrust her on herself and she needed time for readjustment.

A woman in the forties had attacks of hyperchlorhydria and abdominal pain for which I could find no objective cause. A test meal had been done, but the result was not to hand when I saw her. She was anxious for an X-ray examination to exclude peptic ulcer or appendicitis; this was done with an entirely negative result. I sent the report of this to her doctor who replied: "Last night I learned from the husband that their married life was unhappy—with no children after many years of marriage. There were squabbles and recriminations. I think one need not look farther than this for the cause of the wife's dyspepsia." And with that I quite agree.

The case of Mrs. Browning is historic. As Elizabeth Barrett, her father had imposed an almost oriental seclusion upon her, for he was determined she should not marry—an attitude towards daughters more common in fathers than is generally supposed. She became an invalid and took to her bed until Robert Browning ran away with her, after which she became quite well.

To question a patient in the presence of another member of the family is worse than useless. For instance, it is usually impossible for a girl to reveal her feelings before her mother. It is unwise for the parent to try and force him or herself (it is usually the latter which attempts it) into a child's confidences, for the child instinctively resents such a potent intrusion into his individuality. It is a painful position on both sides, and in these days when girls are in process of acquiring more independence, the tension between a mother and her growing-up daughter is often distressing. I am always sorry for the mother who believes that her daughter tells her everything, and who says: " We're more like two sisters," because I know if I talk to the girl by herself her usual opening remark is " Mother's the limit ! " Sometimes she tries to cover up this feeling of which she is ashamed by excessive fussing over her mother, but sooner or later out comes the truth. In these matters there can be useful co-operation between the general practitioner and the consultant. The former knows the environment and sees both sides in a family difficulty, while patients find it easier to tell their secret to the latter as he is a stranger whom they need not see again. A married woman with children once told me that the real source of her ill-health was a woman friend who was always imploring her to leave home and share her "well of loneliness." I remarked that she had never told her doctor this; she admitted it, and asked how I knew. I pointed out that she had given me her address as No. 12 in a certain road and that her doctor had written to me from No. 10 in the same road. Some things are too difficult to tell a neighbour, even if he is a doctor.

A doctor seeing a case for the first time may occasionally use shock tactics with success. A friend of mine, a general practitioner, was called to see a young lady in a flat. He was shown into the sitting room and noted that while there were no photographs of young men there were many of women, particularly one of a masculine type. When he was ushered into the bedroom he noted a cabinet photograph of the same masculine woman by the bedside. He was told a long and rambling story of pains for which careful physical examination revealed no cause. He then said: "Do you want me to tell you what I think is the cause of your trouble?" "Yes, that is why I sent for you," was the reply. "But some are not strong enough to bear the truth," he went on. "You really want me to tell it to you?" "Yes." "Well" he said, dramatically pointing to the photograph, "*that* is the cause." The patient rose up in her bed: "How *dare* you," she said, "how dare you insult me like that."

My friend said: "I am very sorry. You asked me to tell you what I thought was the matter, and I did so. I can quite understand that having dropped such an appalling brick, you will prefer not to see me again." He rose to go, but before he reached the door the patient called out: "Stop; it's quite true; how did you guess it?"

Is the human race, as it becomes more sensitized, doomed to suffer more and more from these " substitute pains " and phobias ? It might be thought that there is little or no chance for improvement since the emotional factor in man is not only the most primitive but the most unchanging. But such a pessimistic conclusion is far from justified. For the first time in the history of man we have two powerful forces making for improvement (1) an increasing number of investigators remorselessly applying biological methods to the understanding of man's mental processes, and (2) an increasing number in the younger generation who are not content to adopt accepted standards without demur, but who are keenly intent on discovering the truth about themselves and their reactions to their environment. In the general conflagration of the War more rubbish was burned up than has yet been realized in some quarters. The questioning of conventional ideas goes on unceasingly ; many of them have been weighed and found wanting. That there is a crudity and harshness in the attitude of the younger generation is a fact which is frequently lamented by their seniors, but in so far as this is the almost inevitable out- come of a sincere determination to discover the truth, it is merely the rough side of a real advance.

True the motto of the ancient Greek philosophers was " know thyself ", but as can be seen from the fact that this text was frequently inscribed beneath a grinning skeleton, it often became degraded to a mere *memento mori* ; the attitude of asking why a man should boast himself if he is so soon to die. The newer application of the saying is to learn to know oneself so as to make the most of life—to know how to live rather than how to die. The old psychology took the highest types of mental activity that could be discovered, explored these by introspection as far as possible, and built up a system on the basis that man is a reasonable being. We have come to realize that he is nothing of the sort. He is merely in process of becoming reasonable. By the pursuit of a more objective method than introspection we are realizing that a little reason mounts guard perilously and indecisively over a whole mass of emotions and instincts inherited from a far distant past, much as the cerebral cortex of the brain exercises a fluctuating degree of control over the mass of grey matter beneath it. It is only by frank recognition of such facts that the reasonable self can increase its control over the unreasoning self.

For the first time, then, human relationships are being studied objectively, and the results of that investigation are proving disconcerting, because the tearing aside of veils is showing that things are other than we have supposed. But that is a temporary phase, before readjustments have had time to be made. In the past many men found it a painful idea that after all the earth was not the centre of the universe and the sun did not move round it. Does that fact worry anyone to-day? On the contrary has not its acceptance both simplified and expanded our conception of the universe? Last century many men were greatly distressed at the idea that man was not a special creation but was evolved for lower forms. Does it distress us to-day? On the contrary, the evolutionary conception reveals a far greater and more wonderful world than our grandfathers had any idea of. Now it is not man's position in the universe or in the animal kingdom that is being questioned—it is the nature of man himself. For a time this will be painful to a good many; the giving-up of preconceived ideas is often painful, but the result of frank acceptance will be release from many obsessions of fear—the bogy boldly faced is seen for the turnip lantern and white sheet that it is. There will be less sheltering behind disabilities created by imaginary pains when we realize that the source of the pain is within ourselves, and that it originates in a conflict between the instinctive and the reasoning self. As long as people lie to their reasoning selves they are bound to suffer.

Clearly it is psychotherapy and not drugs that are called for in cases of substitute pains. But in the cases of physical pain it is clear that the psychological factor also enters into treatment. It would appear from recent researches that the state of the emotions can very definitely influence the action of the drugs we employ. Herein we find the scientific explanation of the fact that hope is the best of tonics. But an essential factor in hope is faith. The patient must be able to believe in you, in your knowledge, care, and skill. You will have to give good grounds for this faith, and in order to inspire it no aspect of the case must be neglected.

Now organic disease is not so common as we often suppose. The wards of a hospital give the student an erroneous impression on this point, since the cases are specially selected. I have asked various general practitioners what proportion of the patients they see are suffering from functional rather than organic disease ; not one of them placed it at less than 40 per cent, while some put it as high as 75 per cent. That is to say, about half to three-quarters of these patients were, broadly speaking, finding difficulty in adapting themselves to their environment. Clearly the trouble might be due to the environment, but also it might be due to themselves. A disturbing emotion will cause palpitations and a sinking sensation in the stomach. The normal individual recognizes this for what it is worth, the psychoneurotic concludes he has heart disease or a gastric ulcer. This enables him to fulfil his unconscious or subconscious desire to retreat from life and evade his duty as a member of the social organism.

I am not blaming him ; his external environment may, indeed, be difficult to-day. It is not surprising that many people find it hard to adjust themselves to conditions which are changing so rapidly. Moreover, the old sense of security has gone.

The foundations of the psychoneuroses are already fairly clearly known ; the plans on which they are formed are consistent and comparatively few, but the elaborations and resistances which are built up on these plans and foundations are often baffling. Yet with sympathy and encouragement they may often be elucidated and the sufferer greatly helped. Although it is true that difficult and complicated cases of this sort call for specialist treatment, it is equally true that the ordinary doctor who goes about with his eyes open for the psychological aspect of disease will soon find that he can greatly increase his usefulness. He will find the simpler methods of Adler not difficult to acquire and not so time-consuming in practice as some others.

It is clear that in some of the cases that I have related there was a genuine cause for painful feeling ; merely explaining how the emotional cause is producing bad health does not do away with the disagreeable emotion. But it brings it more under the control of the reasoning self—it does away with the terror of the unknown, and the sufferer is able to face the situation with a calmer courage.

The difference between a machine and a living organism such as man lies in this : the more perfect a machine the less adaptable it is ; a small defect in the mechanism may reduce it to impotence. The human organism, on the other hand, can overcome obstacles that one would think must break it and, after all, through those very difficulties achieve something fine.

Sir James Mackenzie neatly defined symptoms as the disturbance of normal reflexes. A normal reflex is certainly purposive, and should be painless. Through a chain of conditioned reflexes we associate ideas and achieve consciousness. This consciousness appreciates that a disturbance of the normal reflex is painful and being still purposive proceeds to investigate the cause of the pain. The dog licks his bite, the burnt child dreads the fire, but from such simple defensive reflexes as these are built up elaborate associations of ideas, until in the process of social evolution certain individuals become set apart to be epicritic on other people's protopathic sensations and to try to rectify these disturbed and there-fore painful reflexes. There is thus no break in the chain between simple reflexes and the evolution of the medical profession. We are, indeed, the last link in a long chain of conditioned reflexes !

THE STYLE OF LIFE

The mental attitude, or what Adler calls the *style of life* is founded in the first five or six years of childhood. From this time onwards the answers to the questions put by life are dictated by an almost automatic response based upon this style. The power motive will express itself quite differently in an only child, the eldest child, the second child, or the youngest child. It is a profound mistake to think that children of the same parents living in the same home have the same environment any more than they have an identical germ plasm. The style of life then formed has later on to adapt itself to three great questions—Society, Occupation, Sex, which we may call the SOS of each individual. Only if he can make suitable adaptations to these three can he be happy and fit. If he is hampered by any structural or functional inferiority in making any of these adaptations there are three possibilities. The result is either (1) overcoming, success, or even triumph; (2) neurosis, psychoneurosis, or psychosis itself; or (3) disease, degeneration, and decay. As Crookshank put it : "For body as for soul, there is the effort that overcomes weakness and leads to strength, the hesitation and *compromise* that means evasion of difficulty and leads to neurosis ; and the despairing *retreat* that entails frank disaster."

The particular aspect I want to stress is the way in which that compromise or retreat almost invariably takes the form of phantasy thinking—the escape into a dream world to compensate for the difficulties of the real one. I should like to illustrate it by one of H. G. Wells's earliest stories—*The Door in the Wall.*

You may remember that story of an outwardly

successful man who had something hidden in his life, a haunting and beautiful memory which made all the interests of worldly life seem dull and tedious to him. His mother died when he was two; his father was a stern, preoccupied lawyer, who gave him little attention but expected great things of him. One day, when he was five years old, he wandered off among some roads in West Kensington. Suddenly in a quiet street a white wall and a green door stood out quite distinctly. He hesitated because he had the clearest conviction that either it was unwise or it was wrong of him, he could not tell which, to yield to this attraction. "Then he had a gust of emotion. He made a run for it lest hesitation should grip him again : he went plump with outstretched hands through the green door and let it slam behind him. And so in a trice he came into the garden that has haunted him all his life." It was an enchanted garden that stretched far and wide, with hills in the distance. "Heaven knows where West Kensington had suddenly got to. And somehow it was like coming home. . . . There was no amazement, but only an impression of delightful rightness, of being reminded of happy things that had in some strange way been overlooked. . . ." Then presently came a sombre dark woman who showed him a book, in the living pages of which he saw himself and all the things that had ever happened to him since he was born, up to the time that he saw himself hovering and hesitating outside the green door in the long white wall, and felt again the conflict and the fear. "And next—next," he insisted and struggled to turn over the page. And as he turned the page he found himself in the long grey street in West Kensington in that chill hour of the afternoon before the lamps are lit.

Again and again he tried to find that door, but the significant thing is that he was never able to find it when he searched. But several times in various crises of his life, he unexpectedly saw the door, but could not stop to enter. Thus when he was driving to Paddington to catch a train for Oxford for a scholarship examination he saw it, dared not stop, and won the scholarship. He said: " My grip was fixing now upon the world. I saw another door opening, the door of my career." While life went successfully and its rewards were adequate he did not see that door. But when he had achieved and become disillusioned by success he found that door and walked through.

Let me tell you the end of the story in the author's own words. " They found his body . . . in a deep excavation near East Kensington Station. It is one of two shafts that have been made in connection with an extension of the railway southward. It is protected by a hoarding, in which a small doorway has been cut for the convenience of the workmen. . . . Did the pale electric lights cheat the rough planking into a semblance of white ? Did the fatal unfastened door awaken some memory ? "

" I am more than half convinced that he had a sense that in the guise of wall and door offered him an outlet, a secret and peculiar passage of escape into another and altogether more beautiful world. At any rate, you will say, it betrayed him in the end. But did it betray him ? There you touch the inmost mystery of these dreamers, these men of vision and imagination. We see our world fair and common, the hoarding and the pit. By our daylight standard he walked out of security into darkness, danger, and death. But did he see like that ? "

To me one of the most interesting things about this parable is that it was written just before the present century, when our ideas on such subjects had hardly taken shape. The boy was a lonely and unhappy child— his first definite step into phantasy took place when he was 5, that is to say when his style of life was just formed. It is the unhappy child who is most the prey of phantasy, as a means of escape. The garden symbolizes such an escape, and you will note that his entrance into it was heralded by a sense of conflict and fear—as all neuroses are. When he tried to turn over the pages of that book of life to read the future, phantasy failed him, as it always does, and he was thrown back into real life. The story particularly insists on the temptation to retreat into phantasy whenever some difficulty presented itself or when some special effort was called for. But when worldly success was attained phantasy had less fascination for him, until that success was found unsatisfying. The final retreat into phantasy was such a gross departure from reality that it brought what seems to us disaster, but was for him an escape. The author's meaning is clear, though the power of his imagination had outrun the then state of our knowledge.

Phantasy, then, represents a retreat, expressing a desire for attainment without effort. Consciously followed for purposes of artistic expression it may add to the beauty and enjoyment of life. Unconsciously or subconsciously adopted as a means of achievement of a desire without effort it always does harm and may lead to serious neuroses. It is quite natural for a child to indulge in phantasy, but unfortunately the attitude adopted towards children in the past, and to a lesser extent even to-day, fosters the carrying of phantasy thinking into adult life. The attitude I refer to is one of implying that all the inevitable limitations and restrictions of childhood will cease when the child is grown up, and at the same time telling him that childhood is the happiest time of life. These statements are glaringly inconsistent, and when their untruth becomes obvious, the disillusionment drives those who are not fairly tough-minded to seek a way of escape. The child must be treated as a reasonable being and a potential adult. Life must be presented to him in terms of reasonable expectation, in language of a kind suited to his stage of development.

Of course to some extent we all live in a world of phantasy. Life would be hardly endurable if our friends treated us with the same frank criticism to our faces that they habitually indulge in behind our backs. We have got to live with ourselves for a long time and it is therefore necessary that we should find ourselves more interesting and charming than others need, who do not see so much of us. We cannot escape from ourselves, but others can and do find respite in our absence.

The clinical importance of phantasy thinking is that it accounts for the undue optimism of some patients and for the imaginary ills of others. The man who tells you that fortunately he has a good constitution, when he is really suffering from all sorts of organic disease, is merely deceiving himself, but it may enable him to bear his ills more hopefully. But don't forget that he is sometimes merely whistling to keep his courage up. To take a simple instance of this method leading to imaginary ills ; a lady aged about forty told me a short time ago that when she was sent to boarding school she loathed it. An only child and not a happy one, she hated the communal life. So she developed a sick headache, and continued to have it until at the end of three weeks she was allowed to go home, never to return to school. The lesson was learned—sick headaches were a way out from things you did not want to do. She has continued to invoke their aid, but has apparently forgotten their unreality; indeed, her handbag is an amusing compendium of remedies. On the very morning she told me this story of her schooldays she had a luncheon engagement which she frankly expected to bore her. I was not surprised that about noon she developed a prostrating headache, which quite incapacitated her from going to that lunch, and she seemed quite unaware that she had, by telling me that story, given herself away completely. I was, further, not at all surprised that later in the day an invitation to dinner and a dance in more agreeable company completely relieved the headache. The power motive, the getting of her own way, was achieved without effort by a retreat.

This power motive, if its normal, healthy expression is barred, may assert itself through weakness. Even an ailing woman can satisfy her power motive by making her husband realize that though he is something in the city, he is nothing much at home !

A girl in the early twenties was admitted to hospital

suffering from various neurotic symptoms and maintaining that she could not see. There was nothing to be found wrong with her eyes. She had been in business and was very happy in her work. One day more help was required in the office and she recommended her younger sister, who was given the work. This younger sister proved herself so much abler than the elder that she was soon promoted over her head and given a larger salary. From that the failure of eyesight dated. The implication of the power motive clearly was "I was only beaten by my younger sister because my eyesight failed", and ultimately by seeming to be blind she became the centre of interest. She was quite cured by psychotherapy, and I was recently told by her doctor that she remained quite well.

Sometimes the neurosis has a more vindictive origin. It is well to note who is being most inconvenienced by the patient's neurotic symptoms. A little further investigation will reveal that the patient has a concealed hostility to this individual. Here there is a real desire to hurt.

A neglected child will generally develop phantasy thinking as a compensation, as in the case of a girl aged 13 with a neuropathic inheritance. Both parents adopted the view that children must be allowed to develop themselves without any interference. But that was merely a cloak for a lack of interest in this child, for the mother was passionately devoted to the younger child, aged 3, who was certainly not allowed to develop without interference. The thirteen-year-old sought importance among her schoolfellows by constantly giving them presents. How she did this out of her pocket-money of 6d. a week was rather dubious, and there was reason to suspect her honesty. One day she told a friend she had lost her purse containing 14s. The next day the purse, now empty, was returned to her through the post. Apparently she had spent the money in some way she did not wish to admit, and posted the empty purse back to herself. All the games she played centred around herself. Once she called together as many of her schoolfellows as she could muster, promising them a wonderful treat. She then produced a toy sixpenny aeroplane which she managed to flutter feebly about while she spun phantastic yarns concerning it. In all this the craving for power and for the limelight is clearly manifested.

The neuroses of the eldest child start from the time when he is dethroned by the arrival of the second. As Adler says: "He uses all the means by which he has hitherto attracted notice. Of course he would like to go the best way about it, to be beloved for his goodness : but this is apt to pass unnoticed when everyone is busied with the newcomer ; and he is then likely to change his tactics. . . . Antagonism, disobedience, attacks on the baby, compel the parents to reconsider his existence. He must have the spotlight on himself. . . . If he finds he can win in a fight, he will become a fighting child : if fighting does not pay, he may lose hope, become depressed and score a success by worrying and frightening his parents, after which he will resort to even more subtle uses of misfortune to gain his end." And we may add that the type of neurosis thus developed is apt to express itself in one of these ways throughout life. But the eldest child—" partly because he often finds himself acting as representative of the parental authority, is normally a great believer in power and the laws." At his public school he is the typical prefect. For the second child, life from the first is more or less of a race ; the first child sets the pace and the second tries to surpass him. It was well-expressed by a little boy of four who cried out, weeping : " I'm so unhappy because I can *never* be as old as my brother." Adler maintains that in later development, the second child is rarely able to endure the leadership of others or to accept the idea of " eternal laws ". He will be much more inclined to believe that there is no power in the world which cannot be overthrown. Beware of his revolutionary subleties. For though it is possible to endanger a ruling power with slander, there are more insidious ways—for instance, by means of excessive praise—you may idealize a man or a method until the reality cannot stand up to it. Both methods are employed in Mark Anthony's oration in *Julius Cæsar*.

The youngest child is apt to be over-indulged or over-stimulated, or both. Adler points out that he is apt to look for a field of activity remote from that of other members of the family, which may be a sign of hidden cowardice. But youngest children tend to be the most successful. If they are not successful in reality, they take care to become so in phantasy. Thus in fairy tales it is always the youngest son who grows rich and marries the princess.

The only child retains the centre of the stage without effort. From the extraordinary care which is lavished upon him he is apt to grow up very cautious. Only children may develop charming manners because from the first they have found this to have a successful appeal. But from the lack of companionship of children of their own age they easily become self-important and precociously adult. Indeed, their frequent inability to make satisfactory contacts with their own generation is one of their besetting difficulties. If pampered they may become tyrannical until the time comes when indulgence can go no further, and then there is open warfare with the parents.

But of all children the adopted child is most prone to phantasy thinking, once he knows the fact. Usually the truth is not revealed to him until his style of life is more or less established. In my experience, his first reaction to being told that he has been adopted is one of unreasoning anger. All the care and devotion he has had go for nothing compared with the feeling that he has been deceived. This is, also, more often than not, quite a severe pain-anger : he had parents and they had no need of him. Why ? Hence the self-exaltation to compensate for the doubts and fears which would tend to a feeling of inferiority. For this reason I am in favour of letting the child realize as soon as possible that he was adopted. The next reaction is phantastic speculation and day-dreaming about his real origin. He usually speedily convinces himself that his parents must have been people of great distinction—phantasy spreads and grows. This particular form of phantasy is apt to occur even apart from the mystery engendered by adoption. For Alexander the Great, even Philip of Macedon was not great enough for a father ; egged on by his mother he at last came to believe that he must be the son of the god Ammon-Ra.

I recently saw a striking example of phantasy thinking in a girl aged 17, who was an adopted child. When told at about the age of ten that she was adopted she developed the exalted parentage phantasy, and tried to walk with a very light step, skimming the ground, because she felt that she was " unlike other people " and rather above the common clay. There was a phase of very emotional dreams at about twelve, and the writing of much poetry for which she showed some aptitude. She also wrote passionate letters (which she did not send) about her love for and visualizing of life with certain sports-heroes and film stars. A maternal longing was also evident as the closing chapter was usually that of the hero-husband tip-toeing into her room for the brief moment allowed by stern doctors and nurses that she might show him the small son nestling in the crook of her arm.

She had great difficulties at school ; she was not good at games or lessons, and did not get on with the other girls. She fluctuated between exaltation and self-abasement, and finally after the holidays refused to return to school on the ground of ill-health. This excuse was also used a great deal to avoid anything she did not want to do. A baby boy was then adopted also and she was very happy in helping to look after him, but soon began to speak of him as " my little son, John ". Later this boy was found to be unsuitable and other arrangements were made for him. This produced more emotional, and now melancholy, verse. Before long she developed definite phantasies of pregnancy.

Phantasy thinking, then, springs from the conflict arising from the difficulty that the individual has in harmonizing his desires with his chances of achievement. I do not think that either Freud, Adler, or Jung's theories are completely satisfactory in explaining the extraordinary reactions which may arise from such conflict. It is unfortunate, even if inevitable, that there should be hostile camps in such matters, for it is clear that each of these schools has some aspect of the truth and that ultimately portions of each theory will be built into the edifice of sound psychotherapy. The Freudian is so occupied with the drains that he can hardly spare time to consider the physical state of his patient, while Jung is apt to retreat into the clouds of mysticism. To the practising physician who is constantly seeing patients troubled in mind, body, or estate, either simply or simultaneously, the more realistic psychology of Adler has an increasing appeal.

Freud's view that infantile sexuality is the basis of all these subterranean conflicts of the mind will almost certainly have to be modified. The conception of the Œdipus complex has been greatly over-stressed, but it remains true that the child's relations to his mother and father are among the most powerful causes of repressions and conflicts later on. His view that the unconscious thinks in symbols is very likely true, but his claim, which has been exaggerated by his followers, that these symbols are the same for everyone is not likely to stand. His insistence on *ambivalence*—i.e. that complexes have a double quality of simultaneous attraction and repulsion, has resulted in a very helpful addition to our knowledge. To take a simple instance—a boy may love and respect his father. " But the father is the source of punishment and the boy is frightened of his anger and galled by his authority. He loves, fears, admires, and dislikes all in one." The mingling of fear and devotion is obvious in most religions.

Adler's view that unsatisfied self-assertion is the main cause of psychoneuroses is also probably true, but does not cover all the facts. But his claim is a sound one that a neurosis is very often adopted as an explanation for lack of success, both to the outside world and to the patient himself. If it were not for this crippling symptom I should have achieved my ambition, is the patient's defence. Look how bravely I bear this incapacity, is his bid for sympathy and admiration.

You will see where Adler departs from Freud—he does not base the neuroses on infantile sexuality and its repressions. The form that the sexual manifestations take in a neurosis is merely determined by the underlying style of life of the individual. I have long felt that it is a mistake to conclude as, Freudians appear to do, that the simple bodily reactions of an infant determine his subsequent adult trends. Surely it is more reasonable to assume that the mental development of an infant is at a stage which is only capable of certain reactions. I do not believe that a man is a miser because he was an anal erotic infant, though they may both be symptoms of an inherent " unwillingness to part ".

Jung's classification of extraverts and introverts has also been very helpful, but its weakness is that it has led to others trying to force individual patients into one or other of these two categories. Whereas the truth is that the vast majority of people are a bit of both. But I regard as most valuable his conception that " it is the general urge of life rather than the particular urge of sex or self-assertion which drives us on towards finer adaptations and fuller satisfactions " (Wells and Huxley). I like his forwardly directed gaze. Let us not look too exclusively at the patient's past but set his mind in the right direction for the future, is the essence of his therapy. And though his idea of a collective unconscious is, in the present state of our knowledge, rather mystical, it is full of suggestion for the future. Briefly he maintains there is a racial as well as an individual unconscious, a store of racial memories laid up in the course of generations, which form the basis of dream-symbolism and of mythology as well. This explains why primitive races, children and psychoneurotics have a similar mentality. You may say that it would also fit in with Freud's claim that the symbols have the same meaning in everyone. But the conception of a group mind, as McDougall called it, is an illuminating one. For is it not clear that there are waves of human thought which arise, one knows not where, but which spread far and wide. Sometimes they can be traced to some powerful individual agency, but more often not. " Who is this Bob, who makes all the girls cut their hair ? " asked an old lady a few years ago. She might well ask, for that " Bob " was a true Time Spirit. The death of so many young men in the War led to a rapid spread of masculinization among girls, to be followed a few years later by a similar but less extreme compensatory feminization among young men. Now there is a return to a more normal orientation. We speak of the Victorian Age as if it were a national phase, but a very little study of the history of other nations will show that there was a very similar state of affairs in them at that time. Like-minded people begin to decorate their rooms in the same style and to admire the same artists and authors at the same time, and that often without any deliberate imitation.

The problem for the psychoneurotic is the same problem which besets us all, but it gives him more difficulty. We all have to adapt the need for self-expression and self-development to the increasing demands of the community in which we live. The same problem confronted unicellular organisms when they became multicellular. The social insects adapted themselves to the needs of the hive or nest by purely instinctive reactions. But for man, with his strongly marked individuality, this is not the road to happiness. His is a far more difficult task, to reconcile his individual needs to the needs of the community. He will find it easier, however, if he realizes that there is no prospect for perfection within his life-time either in his own career or in the civilization of which he forms a part. For we are such a recent and untried development. I like Jeans's simile—take a column the height of Cleopatra's Needle as representing the duration of life on the earth ; then a penny laid on the top would represent on the same scale, the time that prehistoric man has existed, while a postage-stamp on the top of the penny would represent the duration of historic time. Increase the column to the height of Mont Blanc and it would represent the time that astronomers can give us for the total duration of life on the earth.

We are living in the first century that has had any knowledge of the enormous scale on which nature works. It might be thought that this would have a depressing effect on individual activity. But as a matter of fact we do not find, as a rule, that a depressed outlook and a retreat to phantasy thinking is common among those who most appreciate this vast scale. Rather is it among those who centre their attention on themselves and neglect the community. One of the first things we have to help the psychoneurotic to do, after unearthing the cause of his trouble, is to get him to feel that it is worth while to work in the common interest. By doing so, as William Brown says, he may lose some individuality but he will gain in personality. William James put it finely when he said : " For my own part I do not know what the sweat and blood and tragedy of this life mean, if they mean anything short of this. If this life be not a real fight, in which something is eternally gained for the universe by success, it is no better than a game of private theatricals, from which one may withdraw at will. But it *feels* like a real fight—as if there were something really wild in the universe which we with all our idealities and faithfulnesses are needed to redeem ; and first of all to redeem our own hearts from atheisms and fears. . . . Be not afraid of life. Believe that life *is* worth living, and your belief will help create the fact."

II

MYTH, PHANTASY, AND *MARY ROSE*

MYTH, PHANTASY, AND *MARY ROSE*[1]

Towards the end of the last glacial epoch, when civilization was just dawning round the group of Mediterranean lakes, the increasing mildness of the climate wrought an enormous disaster. For the melting ice so raised the level of the ocean that the Atlantic burst through the Pillars of Hercules and flooded these lakes, converting them into an inland sea, overwhelming the inhabitants. Of this there is ample geological evidence. We may justly infer that survivors climbed up on to the higher surrounding ground, for everywhere around that flooded area we find the legend of the Deluge, differing locally according to local experiences. Thus the Greek version differs substantially from the Jewish, which indeed hails from Sumeria. I would suggest that some of those Sumerian survivors, who reached the higher lands, did so by the aid of some primitive raft or boat, accompanied by their domestic animals, and thus gave rise to the story of the Ark.

The first point I wish to make, at any rate, is that behind the myth there is generally a fact mingled with a phantasy. The next is that myth is particularly apt to arise at some time of national danger and distress, when men's imaginations are keenly aroused. Such myths may be more potent when tradition is oral and not written, yet remembering such recent history as the Great War, one hesitates to affirm so much. For in a sceptical age, amid the clamour of the daily press, arose such legends as the Angels at Mons, the Russians pouring from Archangel through England on their way to the Western Front, and Kitchener resurgent from the sea as Kerensky or Korniloff—it mattered little which.

The Greeks were the greatest of myth-makers, just because they had the gift of a supreme literary style, which has ensured the permanence of their legends. But it has been left to the present generation to exhume the historical basis of those myths which had been in existence for 3,000 years. Excavations at Crete, Mycenæ, and Troy have revealed indisputable evidence that the stories of the Greek Heroes symbolize and epitomize the struggles between the older Minoan civilization in the south and the invaders from the north. In this way arose such myths as the Minotaur. The bull was the national symbol of Crete, and the excavation of the palace of Cnossus has revealed his emblems everywhere ; the whole palace is his labyrinth. The Athenians represented him as a cruel monster, demanding every seventh year his toll of Athenian youths and maidens. This merely means that for a time the Cretans levied tribute on the Athenians. The story of the Argonauts represents the efforts of the invading races from the north to trade and colonize along the Dardanelles and up to the Black Sea, which followed the destruction of the Mycenæan civilization of Troy. The fight between Pallas Athene and Poseidon to decide who should be the tutelary deity of Athens has a similar significance, for Poseidon as the Sea King represented the naval power of Crete, and his defeat by Athene symbolizes the waxing of Athenian power.

We must always remember that between the earlier Minoan and Mycenæan civilizations and the classical age of Greece there was a gulf as deep and as dark as that which separates the fall of Rome from modern civilization. In that dark interval, the author or, more probably, authors of the Homeric poems sang of glories they had never seen. That this earlier civilization was of a high grade we have abundant evidence in their palaces, their jewels, and pottery. Their womenfolk wore a costume remarkably like that worn about forty years ago, fitting tightly round the waist, and below this a bell skirt with about five rows of flounces. Their sanitation was admirably modern. But before 1000 B.C. all this had perished, and when the author of the *Odyssey* describes the return of Ulysses to his ancestral home we read of his faithful dog lying on a dung-heap before the front door of his palace ; he tells us that Nausicaa, a King's daughter, was doing her own laundry work. The people of Homer's time had no idea of the style in which their predecessors had lived ; they figured them as living under the simple conditions that they themselves knew, merely exaggerating the size of things. Just so Daisy Ashford in *The Young Visiters* pictured a peer living in " compartments " in the Crystal Palace, with strawberry ices for staple diet. The imaginings of primitive people and of childish minds are remarkably similar. But the important thing for us to realize is that these myths are based on facts and distorted by phantasy, just as the stories children make up are based on their own experience, similarly distorted. It has been well said that the dream is the myth of the individual life, and the myth is the dream of the national life. Certain it is that the dream assumes special intensity and significance when conflict occurs within the individual, just as the myth most readily springs out of national conflict.

Phantasy is a day-dream, arising like the ordinary dream out of the unconscious and, like it, is often aroused by internal conflict, expressing unfulfilled desires. " Man is essentially an image-maker, but it is his human prerogative. In most animals, who act from what we call instinct, action follows on perception mechanically with almost chemical swiftness and certainty. In man the nervous system is more complicated ; perception is not instantly transformed into reaction ; there seems to be an interval for choice. It is just in this momentary pause between perception and reaction that our images, i.e. our imaginations, our ideas, in fact our whole mental life is built up. We do not immediately react, i.e. we do not immediately get what we want, so we figure the want to ourselves—we create an image. If reaction were instant, we should have no image, no representation, no art, no theology. In Greek mythology we have enshrined the images fashioned by the most gifted people the world has ever seen, and these images are the outcome, the reflection of that people's unsatisfied desire " (Jane Harrison).

It follows that in works of imagination we are very likely to find traces of the unconscious mind of the author, and that these are likely to appeal to a wide audience in proportion to the extent they resume and symbolize things of universal experience. Some of them, like Stevenson's *Dr. Jekyll and Mr. Hyde*, as we shall see in another chapter, are admitted to have originated in a dream. This particular story shows another characteristic of a dream—the condensation of two characters into a single personality. For as I shall detail in a later chapter Dr. Jekyll is a composite portrait of two actual and recognizable individuals.

But I think that phantasy from the unconscious is a more common origin of imaginative works than dreams. Anthony Trollope did his own reputation as a novelist enormous harm by representing his writing as a purely business task as much part of his daily routine as his breakfast. Much of his work is, in my opinion, of too subtle a character to make this likely ; but the public resentment of such a mechanical origin was based on a sound if unrecognized feeling that this is not the way that literature is produced.

E. F. Benson describes the way his unconscious dictated his writing thus : " I can still taste the relish of coming in out of a wet November evening, knowing that they (the characters in my tale) would be waiting in my sitting-room for me, and presently, with Out displayed on my door, I would immerse myself and see what they proposed to do. For, indeed, if the book, in my biased judgment was going well, it seemed as if the persons I was writing about took charge of their own manœuvres, while I, who held the pen, did little more than record their independent action. Often I would have planned, even with detail, what I meant to do with them, only to find that they had planned and now dictated something else. Of course, it was really my brain that was doing it all but, so I imagine, some part of it, not quite identical with my conscious self, took control. And when this seemed to be happening I was careful to distract the more superficial cells. I gave them cigarettes to smoke, occasionally played them a tune on the piano ; did anything to divert them so that they should not interfere with what was going on below.

". . . On these evenings, when the mysterious workman was in possession, I took pains not to disturb him, and . . . forebore to question him about his plans while I sedulously amused my conscious self . . . so that, diverted and occupied, it should not meddle. Sometimes it insisted on interfering, and when I got to work again would make itself so importunate that its ally, always sensitive and touchy, would shut up altogether and refuse to make any more plans.

"On more fortunate evenings I could quite hold the interfering partner's attention. . . . Swiftly passed those auspicious hours, but at the end the dictating voice ceased, even in the middle of a sentence, and it was long past midnight, and there were a dozen sheets of paper covered with writing, and I, tired and sleepy and wonderfully satisfied. I just arranged the sheets, shuffled off to bed, and slept the perfect dreamlessness of fatigue.

". . . Again and again have I cudgelled my brains as I dressed, in the effort to remember what I had written, and been totally unable to recollect it, so that I would read it over with surprised interest. Often these subconscious scribblings required correction and

127

trimming, for sentences would be unbalanced and phrases needed the file or called for recasting, but the substance and general outline invariably met with the approval of my conscious self, who realized over his eggs and bacon that he had not and could not have devised the stuff. He might not think very highly of it, but he always passed it on those occasions when he had nothing to do with it."

That novelists may fail to recognize the source of inspiration in their own unconscious was demonstrated to me by a friend of mine, a woman novelist. To anyone who knew her upbringing and her family environment her reaction to them is sufficiently obvious in her stories, but she herself indignantly and, I believe, sincerely denies that any of her characters are drawn from life. She wrote to her sister saying that she hoped she did not think that a certain character was her portrait, as had been alleged. Her sister very neatly replied : " My dear, I am much too conceited to see myself in any of your stories." Yet to me the portrait seemed lifelike.

Schubert said : " My music is the product of my pain—and that which has cost me the most pain to produce the world seems to have the most pleasure in listening to." His " Unfinished Symphony " is an obvious example of this, and the fact that it is unfinished expresses his failure to resolve the conflict it describes. Lord Baldwin's striking description of " the drum-taps of destiny " in Beethoven's fifth symphony illustrates the same idea, but here the composer escaped from the mocking goblin music of the third movement into the triumphant finale.

For the physiologist, then, imaginative works of art spring from a failure of conditioned reflexes to achieve their purpose, and for the psychologist they often express internal conflict. They are a house of defence. I have said elsewhere that the difference between a machine and a man lies in this. The more complicated the former is the more completely can it be arrested by a trivial defect, while a man confronted by obstacles which may appear overwhelming and crushing to the outsider, can turn them to advantage and make something fine out of his very difficulties. The satisfied man is not likely to be an artist. Morley Roberts has openly declared that his novels spring from dissatisfaction. The old wish, "Oh that mine enemy would write a book," assumes a new meaning now that the psychologist has provided us with a key which unlocks many things which the author imagines are safely hid.

I think this method of approach to an author is going to make literary criticism a more living thing. It will only be resented by those who like to think that a genius springs like Pallas Athene, full-grown from the head of Zeus. This, to my mind, was the secret of the opposition to Clemence Dane's play *Will Shakespeare*. For she represented Shakespeare as a man growing and learning by his very mistakes. Which, whether he was Bacon or not, he most certainly must have done. The genius learns from his mistakes and turns them to the triumphant advantage of himself and others ; the fool learns nothing from them, and merely comes to think the universe has a grudge against him.

The old Stoic philosophy had the root of the matter in it for, as Gilbert Murray tells us: "Stoicism does not really make reason into a motive force. It explains that an impulse of physical or biological origin rises into the mind, prompting to some action, and then reason gives or withholds its assent." Unfortunately reason is not always a sufficiently powerful censor. H. G. Wells put it forcibly when he said : "The substance of man is ape still. He may carry a light in his brain, but his instincts move in the darkness. Out of the darkness he draws his motives."

The new psychology is in effect based upon the old biological law of recapitulation. Every animal has to climb up his own genealogical tree, and the higher he climbs the more difficult this becomes. Every step in development demands some break with the past. If we retain some atavistic trait this step may be impeded or impossible. Such traits may be physical or psychical in character. To see things as they are is the task of growing up. To a certain extent we all tend to grow up in patches. Sir Arthur Keith has recently made the profound remark that the tendency to carry youthful characteristics into adult life has played a large part in the evolution of human races. He was speaking at the time of the variations which differentiated man from the anthropoids but, like many of his remarks, it has a much wider application. This power of carrying youthful characters into adult life turned an ape into a man, but just as it may be a source of strength, so it may become a besetting weakness. Its function is to maintain a plasticity out of which higher characteristics can be moulded ; its weakness is that the childish or primitive attitude may persist. Failure to adapt physically leads to disease ; failuie to adapt psychically lies at the root of much unhappiness. This failure may express itself in one of several forms of atavistic thinking.

Thus under stress of emotion there may be, in effect, a return to the savage's belief in magic. The savage always attributes death to murder or magic. A few years ago a lady had the pleasure of paying £100 damages to her doctor for alleging that he had murdered her husband. A little appreciation of the reality principle would have convinced her that, putting it at its lowest, there are good and sufficient reasons why a doctor would not murder a patient who was a distinguished baronet. That is not the way practices are built up or maintained. The poor lady in the grief of her bereavement reverted to a primitive method of thinking. As recently as Tudor times allegations of poisoning followed every royal death, except where that death was clearly due to the executioner's axe. Well, we have outgrown that stage.

Another atavistic belief is in the omnipotence of thought. The savage believes he has only to want a thing badly enough for it to become true. In the same way the psychoneurotic easily convinces himself that what he wants has come true, and closes his eyes to anything which would conflict with that idea. Thus he loses touch with reality.

But most commonly we see atavism in the fixation of some childish attitude of mind. What is normal for one epoch of life is abnormal for another. Let me deal with father fixation first. At a certain stage the father represents the idea of omnipotence to the child. " What do you think God is like ? " said one little girl to another. " Rather like my daddy," said the other. " Like *my* daddy you mean," was the indignant reply. It is hardly necessary to say that this is a transient phase. The inability of most fathers to live up to such an ideal is too obvious. What is the reaction of a psychoneurotic who has to face this failure ? He very often will not give it up, but concludes that his alleged parent is really not his father. Only someone very much greater could have begotten such a wonderful being as himself. In milder degrees such phantasies are quite common. Take one which came to my notice. A foundling grew up to be a gardener and married one of the servant-maids of the house. Their child was given a very good start by her employers, who thought highly of her. He rose to a successful position in the City, and then became convinced that his unknown grandfather must have been a very distinguished person. He pitched on the most aristocratic family in the neighbourhood where his childhood was spent, convinced himself that one of them was his grandfather, and to this day actually uses their family crest as his own !

Compare George Meredith's deliberate mystification about his own origin, although he draws a picture of his tailor grandfather as the " Great Mel " in his novel *Evan Harrington.*

The next stage in evolution was the father as " the old man of the tribe ". Fixation at this stage of thought produces a more unpleasant reaction. For the old man of the tribe excited jealousy and rebellion. This jealousy is often seen and may become intense. It is not too much to say that an important factor in exciting the outbreak of the Great War was the jealousy between a megalomaniac father and a degenerate son—surely the most disastrous effect of a reversion to the cave-man's way of thinking that the world has ever seen. Minor degrees of such reactions are quite common, and in many a household there is a veiled and often comparatively harmless conspiracy of the mother and sons against the father, by means of which the old man is successfully fooled.

There is another interesting aspect of the father-complex. Said Voltaire : "God made man in His own image, and man hastens to return the compliment." The disappearance from theology of an angry, jealous Jehovah who had to be placated, and the disuse of the term " God-fearing " as a term of approbation, I attribute to the almost complete disappearance of the autocratic, overbearing Victorian father. His maleficent influence can still be seen, however, in the psycho-neuroses of his unfortunate offspring.

Mother fixation is another fruitful cause of psycho-neurosis. Dependence on the mother, normal during a certain stage of life, becomes pathological if it persists as the child grows up. Even if he escapes from it, such an individual merely seeks a substitute.

It really seems that the only happy marriage possible for a man in the toils of this complex is with a maternal cousin. Such a union may be very successful ; Charles Darwin was an illustrious example of this. The death of the mother does not diminish the fixation ; rather, it increases it by attaching to it an immortal memory. I have encountered painful examples of this in my practice, and it is well portrayed in Middleton Murry's novel, *The Things we are*. The cardinal feature has been described as " an inability to adapt to situations requiring any independence of thought and action ", but it has many repercussions. Mother fixation is usually accompanied by more or less of that hostile reaction to the father I have referred to.

Sooner or later any fixation leads to regression. Life cannot be static ; either we must progress or regress. Some animals evade the struggle for existence by degeneration. Regression is the psychological parallel which attends the attempt to escape from reality. Involution is the physical change in old age which brings a mental change with it—that senile obstinacy which, as Clifford Allbutt said, " seems like mellow wisdom to its possessor." But regression is a psychological change which may occur at any age ; it leads to a more and more infantile mode of thinking as the retreat from reality increases. As a beautiful description in literature of regression I would instance Stevenson's *Will o' the Mill*.

With which lengthy preamble I hope I have sufficiently cleared the way for a discussion of *Peter Pan* and *Mary Rose*. But here I may have to meet the objection that Barrie is impossible on account of his sentiment. I can quite understand that to youth of the War and post-War periods sentiment is abhorrent. I can even understand why Epstein appeals to them, though not to me. Let me illustrate my point from a rather striking letter which appeared in the *New Statesman* : " The dominant characters of subhuman and of the lower level of human nature have been displayed with the insight and force of genius in the Epstein Rima. A very large section of the public look at Nature through the rose-tinted glasses of a pseudo-romantic sentiment. They visit the bird sanctuary expecting to see their vision charmingly embodied, as it actually is in the statue of Peter Pan across the water. They are confronted with the less pleasing truth seen by Mr. Epstein's naked eye. Disappointed and shocked, they exclaim against the ugliness and falsehood of his work. But the spirit of Nature he has expressed with unforgettable power ; and it is well that we should all be compelled to look at it in the face of Rima." That is the reason for the spirit which rejects sentiment, and it is chiefly the outcome of the War, the spirit that recognizes how thin is the veneer of civilization. But it is sufficient for my purpose this evening if you will admit the view that sentiment " is an intensely human emotion, intimately linked with our self-pity, our vanity, our impossible aspirations ", for then you must also admit that if Barrie's sentiment enables us to understand more of the workings of the mind, especially at the subconscious level, he is worth studying for the light he throws on these problems.

If you go on to urge that Barrie's sentiment is not sincere, I should be inclined to agree with you on occasions, but would claim that the victim of a fixation is apt to hide his real feelings behind dramatized emotions. For that Barrie was the subject of an intense mother fixation is sufficiently obvious ; his biography of his mother, *Margaret Ogilvy*, proclaims it aloud. He even published his first articles under her maiden name, adopting the pseudonym " Gavin Ogilvy ". The child that " might have been " in *Dear Brutus* is called Margaret. It was his mother as a child that appealed most to his childish imagination. He says : " I soon grow tired of writing tales unless I can see a little girl, of whom my mother has told me, wandering confidently through the pages. Such a grip has her memory of her girlhood had upon me since I was a boy of six "— the age that fixes the style of life. And the consequence of this mental attitude is seen in his statement that " The horror of my boyhood was that I knew a time would come when I also must give up games " ; it leads him to the astonishing remark: " Nothing that happens after we are 12 matters very much." In praise of Robert Louis Stevenson he says: "He was the spirit of boyhood tugging at the skirts of this old world of ours and compelling it to come back and play."

His mother said she would have " liked fine " to have been the mother of a great explorer, of Carlyle, or Gladstone. Evidently her maternal instinct was intensely strong, but it is the tragedy of such forceful personalities that they defeat their own desires by holding the son

in eternal bondage. Said Barrie to her of his books—
" Mother, what a way you have of creeping in."

When Peter Pan came flying back home he found the
nursery window barred, but for Barrie that window
was always open, and therein he found his retreat.
From his books and plays one can construct the life-
history of the genus Peter Pan, that elusive creature
who wanted Wendy for a mother, firmly declining any
more adult relationship. You will find his earliest
phases in *Sentimental Tommy*—the boy who at the
age of six had the imaginative and imitative faculty
so developed and had such a craving for sympathy that
he simulated at one time a reformed prisoner and at
another an epileptic. " His pity was easily aroused for
persons in distress, and he sought to comfort them by
shutting their eyes to the truth as long as possible."
In spite of this equipment for becoming a successful
doctor, he firmly determined on reaching the fa al
age of 12 not to grow up any further. The next phase
of the boy forced to go on with life while never attaining
manhood is to be found in *Tommy and Grizel*—not at all
a good novel, but an enlightening book. Tommy, apt
at simulating emotion, became a popular author by the
time he was 22, though his book was such as to lead
Grizel to say: " If writing makes you live in such an
unreal world, it must do you harm." The whole book
seems to have been written to express contempt for the
artistic temperament. But perhaps we have the key
at the end, where Barrie says, " Have I been too cunning,
or have you seen through me all the time ? Have you
discovered I was really pitying the boy who was so fond
of games that he could not with years become a man,
telling nothing about him that was not true, but doing
it with unnecessary scorn in the hope that I might goad
you into crying ' Come, come, you are too hard on
him '."

On another page he says of Tommy : " He was still
a boy, trying sometimes to be a man, and always when
he looked round he ran back to his boyhood as if he saw

it holding out its arms to him and inviting him to come back and play. He was so fond of being a boy that he could not grow up. In a younger world where there were only boys and girls, he might have been a gallant figure."

Then note how he comports himself when faced by the next step : "If she would only have let him love her hopelessly. Oh, Grizel had only to tell him there was no hope and then how finely he would behave. He saw himself passing through life as her very perfect knight." But when he found himself in danger of being accepted he was appalled. He knew that he had reached the critical moment in her life and his, and that if he took one step forward he could never again draw back. He had a passionate desire to remain free. "He heard the voices of his little gods screaming to him to draw back." In spite of himself he becomes engaged, breaks it off, and then writes a touching book called *Unrequited Love* which, of course, gains him all the sympathy and her all the odium for the rupture. The same capacity for describing emotions he does not feel was evinced in another of his touching books called *The Wandering Child*—a reverie about a little boy that was lost : "His parents find him in a wood singing joyfully to himself because he thinks he can now be a boy for ever ; and he fears that if they catch him they will compel him to grow into a man, so he runs farther from them into the wood, and is running still, singing to himself because he is always to be a boy." But when Tommy was reading aloud one of the most exquisite chapters about the lost child, a real child in the room would not keep quiet, whereupon our sentimental author jumped up and promptly boxed that child's ears. No wonder that in a moment of self-recognition he said: "I seem to be different from all other men. There seems to be a curse upon me." There was—the curse of mother fixation, which held him back in the chains of phantasy, and which may make an artist, but never a man. Aaron Latta said to Tommy: "Your

136

mother was a wonder at make-believe. But she never managed to cheat herself. That's where you sail awa' e'en from her." I have merely put extracts from this book together ; they require no comment ; they seem to me a complete descripton of the genus Peter Pan between the ages of 20 to 30.

Peter Pan in middle age is to be found in *The Little White Bird*. I do not feel that it is permissible to treat the writings of an author as if they were strictly auto-biographical, but it is pretty clear from the time this book was written Barrie's imagination was carried to a much higher flight. Apart from the sketches of life in Thrums I do not think that any of his work up to this point has much chance of immortality. But from this point onwards something new came into his books, or rather, his plays, for he wrote no more stories after this, finding the stage a better medium for his genius. And we know that something new came into his life at this time, for he found in Kensington Gardens some children who influenced his whole outlook. For the first time he ceased to look back regretfully on his own childhood and delighted in the next generation—the only hope for the middle-aged. The man or woman who looks back becomes, like Lot's wife, a pillar of salt— the symbol of unavailing tears. In this book we see Peter Pan the elder as the lonely bachelor who, at his club, is called the confirmed spinster. He is, by the way, supposed to be a soldier—a pathetic attempt at compensation. He is also determined to dodge being called a whimsical fellow, but comes " agitatedly to the fear there may be something in it ".

We next see him grown a little older, as Mr. Coade in *Dear Brutus*. He is described as " old, a sweet pippin of a man with a gentle smile for all ; he must have suffered much, you conclude incorrectly, to acquire that tolerant smile." " His study walls are lined with boxes which contain dusty notes for his great work on the Feudal System, the notes many years old, the work, strictly speaking, not yet begun. He still speaks at times of finishing it, but never of beginning it." " I have often thought, Coady," he says to his wife, " that if I had had a second chance I should be a useful man instead of a nice lazy one." But the second chance shows him still busy with evasion, the " whimsical fellow " who faintly hears the Pan pipes and tries to imitate their music. Allied to Mr. Coade is Mr. Morland in *Mary Rose*—it is interesting to note, by the way, that the same actor was selected to play both these parts. Of all this group Morland alone achieves paternity, and he makes some sort of effort to shoulder responsibility. Still, he says of himself: " I have been occupied all my life with such little things—all very pleasant, I cannot cope, I cannot cope—" And he says his epitaph should be : " In spite of some adversity he remained a lively old blade to the end."

The last scene of all which ends this strange eventful history is to be found also in *Dear Brutus*. Here we meet Lob who, grown inevitably out of these others, retreats from death. And note his Puckish attitude to life : " Those things most please me which turn out preposterously." But of Lob, Puck, Robin Goodfellow, call him what you will, two different views are possible. The harshest one is that of a creature who does not appear to sympathize with man's struggle to break his chains. He collects a number of people who are failures, pushes them out into the enchanted wood of the second chance, and chuckles at the thought that they must fail as surely the second time as they did the first. He laughs : " You'll fail, you'll fail ; I said you would. Destiny and circumstance are too strong for you." And thus he excuses his own failure.

The gentler view may be deduced from Barrie's own description of Lob as he stands there after sending them out into the wood for their second chance : " Quivers of rapture are running up and down his little frame." His glee is paramount ; but his experiment suggests a wistful belief still in some transmuting power, in the light of which the individual can make something out of his second chance. I think he had hopes of Dearth, the artist, who in the wood becomes also a man, once he has found his daughter there. Witness his care for the things she is to see and know : he winces at her growing up, but he is ready to face it. Dearth alone justifies his second chance and makes good ; all the others remain as they were. For he alone had been the victim of circumstance ; the others failed again because they were what they were.

Lob, though so old, is still childish. Crossed in his wishes he creeps under the table, bursts into tears, crying out: " It isn't good for me not to get the thing I want." But he has learned, I think, something from life—an almost prankish benevolence, an uncanny insight into the wonder of youth and joy, of pity and tenderness. And this is Peter Pan grown old ; this is the final stage of the boy who would not accept a man's burden. And there are many such ; indeed, there are not many who can truthfully say: " When I became a man I put away childish things." Lob retreats from death, I have said, and is it not the Lob spirit of Barrie himself which will achieve immortality ? The only time I had the pleasure of meeting Barrie I mentioned the idea that Lob was Peter Pan grown old. He said : "That's good ; how did you find it out ? " I replied : " My wife told me." " She must be a remarkable woman," was his comment.

I want specially to stress the whole genesis of Peter Pan from mother fixation. You will remember that a little girl in a magenta frock and a white pinafore appears in front of the curtain before the play begins and bobs a curtsey to the audience. She appears several times in an inconsequent kind of way in the play, remarks that she is a married woman herself, and at the end flies off on a broomstick. She used to be called the author of the piece on the programmes, but this has now been dropped. Now Barrie told his mother she was really the author of all his books, and the closing sentence of *Margaret Ogilvy* is to the effect that he would always remember her as " a little girl in a magenta frock and a white pinafore who comes towards me through the long parks, singing to herself". Note that Grizel in *Sentimental Tommy* is similarly attired.

At the conscious level Barrie can speak of " a man I am very proud to be able to call my father ", but that is about the only time he speaks of him at all, although he talks at length about his maternal grandfather. But in Peter Pan there is persistent lampooning of the father. For several years the part of Mr. Darling and Captain Hook were taken by the same actor, as if to stress the fact that the Pirate King of the phantasy represented the father. So that there shall be no mistake about this Michael says when he sees his father on his return : " Why, he's not nearly so big as the pirate I killed on the ship." Then note the entirely different reaction of the father and the mother to the loss of the children ; the mother is heart broken, but the father actually gets satisfaction out of his penance of riding to the city in the dog-kennel. Mother fixation always involves some degree of hostile reaction to the father, as I have already said.

If Peter Pan is the boy who wouldn't grow up, Mary Rose is the girl who wasn't allowed to grow up. I think in some respects *Mary Rose* is Barrie's greatest work. To deal with it fully is impossible ; it would be too like Archbishop Whately's edition of Bacon's *Essays*—pages of obvious commentary for every one of Bacon's terse, telling sentences. For it seems to me one of the completest expositions of the working of the unconscious mind to be found in contemporary literature. As Dr. Constance Long said : " A universal problem is dramatized [in it], and one which is of supreme importance in the development of each individual."

The story begins near the end, with the return of Mary Rose's soldier son to the ancestral home, now emptied of everything but a scared caretaker and a ghost. And as he dreams by the fire, the lives of those to whom as a child he meant so much rise up again before him and re-enact their story in its old setting.

Mr. and Mrs. Morland cannot realize that Mary Rose is growing up. They are in love with her as a child, and child she must remain for their delectation. When Mrs. Morland realizes that Simon is in love with her daughter and she with him, it is a terrible shock, but Mr. Morland simply won't face it. He thinks Simon is expecting his usual tip, until his wife says : " James, you may as well be told bluntly ; it isn't your fiver that Simon wants, it is your daughter." And Mary Rose, still bound in the chains of a father fixation, says : " Daddy, I am so awfully sorry this has occurred." While she says to Simon : " It isn't you I'm thinking of ; it is father, it is poor father—Oh, Simon, how could you ? Isn't it hateful of him, Daddy." Barrie does not fail to show that, charming as the home life of the Morlands was, it was a charm that belonged to the nursery, and was fatal to due development of character.

And now Simon had to be told of a strange event when Mary Rose was about 12 years old ; of a visit to the Hebrides, to a small island " that likes to be visited ". There seemed to be nothing very particular about the island, unless, perhaps, that it was curiously complete in itself—a sort of miniature land. Thus Mr. Morland described it. Here Mary Rose suddenly disappeared for twenty days, and as suddenly reappeared, ignorant that she had been out of the world at all. I think there is no doubt that Barrie symbolizes thus a retreat into the world of phantasy at the dawn of puberty. Just when the need came for a more adult adjustment she retreated into a day-dream, as might be expected in a child so secluded from life. And the world of phantasy is curiously complete in itself—a microcosm. An island implies isolation. The technical psychological term for this retreat is a " fugue ". I do not know whether the man who coined this apt term meant simply that it was a flight, or whether he was also thinking of its musical connotation, which involves a repetition of the flight. Certain it is that the individual who once experiences a fugue is likely to have another. The neuroses of the

War have forced us to recognize the reality of such fugues, but they existed before the War. I saw an example in the South African War but, of course, failed to recognize its significance. Rebecca West has described such an incident with delicate insight in *The Return of the Soldier*.

And then comes a delicious piece of dialogue :

"SIMON : 'You told no one?'
"Mr. MORLAND : 'Several doctors.'
"SIMON : How did they explain it?'
"Mr. MORLAND : 'They had no explanation for it, except that it never took place.'"

I appreciate this sly hit at the pre-War materialism of my profession. We had no explanation of the symptoms of our neurotic patients except that they never happened. Phobias, obsessions, fugues! Nonsense! Rubbish! Buck up ; pull yourself together. That was all. Very satisfactory to the doctor, no doubt, who thanked God he was a sensible fellow. But perhaps it was a less satisfactory attitude for the patient.

But to return to our story. Simon asks : " It has had no effect on her, at any rate." Mr. Morland replies : " None whatever—and you can guess how we used to watch." But Mrs. Morland had more insight, and she replies : " Simon, I am very anxious to be honest with you. I have sometimes thought that our girl is curiously young for her age—as if—you know how just a touch of frost may stop the growth of a plant and yet leave it blooming ; it has sometimes seemed to me as if a cold finger had once touched my Mary Rose." There is the penalty of living in a life of phantasy—it is a retreat from life that checks growth.

And now an interesting thing happens. The island had completely faded from Mary Rose's memory. But her engagement makes a new demand on her to grow up, and she remembers her island and wishes to revisit it. The infantile personality faced with a new situation always wants to retreat. It is the fashion to despise

Dickens to-day, but his quick eye for the abnormal in appearance and behaviour enabled him to describe some diseases before the medical profession recognized them. And you may remember that he describes Dr. Manette in the *Tale of Two Cities* as a sufferer from fugues. Whenever he was faced with a difficult situation he retreated from it to become a prisoner in the Bastille again.

In the next act we are on the island ; Simon and Mary Rose have been married for four years ; their baby son is 2¾ years old. Cameron, who rows them over, is a student at Aberdeen in term time ; in the vacation a boatman, or a ghillie, or anything you please, to help pay his fees. He tells them weird stories of the island. Cameron is a delightful character—a fine blend of the intuitive and the rational ; in the Hebrides, full of phantasy, in Aberdeen the classic and philosopher. One may compare him, as Dr. Crichton Miller has done, with the double personality of William Sharp, who, severely intellectual when writing under his own name, found an outflow for his phantasies under the pen-name of Fiona Macleod, inspiring Rutland Boughton to compose *The Immortal Hour*. No nation has ever equalled the Scots in driving phantasy and intellect in double harness. No wonder it has enabled them to achieve greater things than any other Celtic race. The Irish drive them tandem, phantasy leading and repeatedly bolting. Many of you have probably seen *Juno and the Paycock*—a terrible picture of the tragedies that result from phantasy predominating in the Irish character. There, mother love, the first spiritual value to emerge from the slime, appears as the only genuine and beautiful emotion. And to my mind *The Playboy of the Western World* is another picture of the ludicrous disaster that phantasy wreaks on the Irish temperament. As for the Welsh, they appear to harmonize the conflict between the intuitive and the rational largely by means of what Mr. Winston Churchill euphemistically calls " terminological inexactitudes ".

While they are preparing to leave the island the mysterious call again comes for Mary Rose. Note that it comes at a time when they have to return to the business of life, and their baby has just reached the age when the development of his own character should begin. Again Mary Rose retreats into phantasy—she vanishes from real life as though she had never been.

I wonder if Barrie was influenced in this conception by *Kilmeny*, the poem by Hogg, the Ettrick shepherd. For here, too, is the story of a girl who vanishes for seven years, returns for a month, and then disappears for ever.

When the next act begins, twenty-five years have passed. Mr. and Mrs. Morland are engaged in just the same pleasant, trivial round of life; but they are old and grey now. Mary Rose has been all but forgotten by her father; but her mother says a little tremulously: "I suppose it is all to the good that as the years go by the dead should recede farther from us . . . we have to live in the present for a very little longer. . . . Even if we could drag her back I think it would be a shame." Simon enters, just promoted to be a captain in the Navy—full of delight at his good luck. He, too, has almost forgotten Mary Rose. And at that very moment they have news of her return. She is approaching the house; Simon had seen her at the station and failed to recognize her. Divided between fear and joy they prepare to receive her, and then she enters, just the same as she was twenty-five years ago. She leaps towards her mother in the old impulsive way, but the vanished years step in between them, as an impassable barrier. "What is it?" she keeps saying; "Tell me, tell me." She rushes to the nursery, expecting to find her son, Harry, still there as a baby. But he ran away to sea years ago, and has vanished from their ken. Moreover, he would be a man of nearly twenty-eight by now. Thomas Hardy himself could not have conveyed more vividly a sense of the impermanence of all things human than has Barrie in this scene.

To me it seems that one of the most poignant moments

in the play is Mr. Morland's obvious distress at her return, which finds expression in his cry: " Do you think she should have come back ? " On this Dr. Constance Long commented thus : " For the infantile character nothing that disturbs serene existence *ought* to happen. There ought to be no irrational occurrences, no sex problems, no revolution, and no death, and, most of all, no resurrections. For such, all ought to happen according to the wish—an end that can only be fictitiously accomplished through phantasy."

You will remember that Bernard Shaw made the various powers-that-be quite willing for Joan of Arc to be canonized so long as it was quite understood that she was dead and in no danger of resurrection.

After a lapse of twenty-five years Mr. Morland did not really want his once-beloved daughter back. Time marches on relentlessly, and the ranks close up as casualties occur. Were the dead to return they would find their places filled, and a disaster greater than death would be enacted, as in the case of Mary Rose. Deep within us, however unwillingly, we must say with Swinburne :

> " We thank with brief thanksgiving,
>   Whatever Gods may be,
>   That no life lives for ever,
>   That dead men rise up never ;
>   That even the weariest river
>   Winds somewhere to the sea."

With Morland's forlorn cry still sounding in our ears the scene fades away, and we are back in the dismantled room, where Harry, the soldier son, is staring wide-eyed into the fire. He tells the caretaker as she returns : " Things of the far past—things that I knew naught of —they came crowding out of their holes and gathered round me ; I saw them all so clear than I don't know what to think." He asks questions about the ghost and gathers that it is Mary Rose, his dead mother, who haunts the house ; seeking, seeking continually for something. He realizes that she is searching for him, but for him as a child, and he says grimly : " There are worse things than not finding what you are looking for ; there is finding them so different from what you had hoped." And when he is left alone again the ghost of Mary Rose appears. He realizes that she has taken the knife he left lying about. Here we have the symbol of the all-powerful mother who would keep the man as a child and rob him of the power he had painfully acquired. " While it is in his mother's hands he is defenceless ; his individuality is in danger of being killed." (Constance Long).

In *The Little White Bird* we find so many germs of Barrie's later work as to justify my statement that it marks a new development in him. Herein we read : " The only ghosts, I believe, who creep into the world are dead young mothers, returning to see how their children fare. What is saddest about ghosts is that they do not know their child. They expect him to be just as he was when they left him. . . . Poor passionate soul, they may even do him an injury. . . . How could the pretty young mother know that the grizzled interloper was the child of whom she was in search ? " Harry had escaped from the home that would always have been a nursery into the world of reality ; whereas his mother had escaped into a world of phantasy. And note that he had escaped by the apple tree in which Mary Rose was wont to hide. Here again the symbolism is clear, for that apple tree first appeared in the human drama in the Garden of Eden.

You will remember that Mr. Morland wanted to cut down that apple tree—the typical senile way of dealing with all difficulties that the tree of life has introduced into the world. Repress it, deny its very existence, is the cry of the old—it cumbereth the ground.

Harry tries to comfort the ghost and makes her quote her own words : " The loveliest time of all will be when he is a man and takes me on his knee, instead of my taking him on mine "—an example, as Dr. Crichton

Miller says, of our fancied adjustments, those we never succeed in making. For when Mary Rose sits on her son's knee she begins to talk baby talk, i.e. she regresses more and more to an infantile personality. Harry breaks out : " How should the likes of me know what to do with a ghost that has lost her way on earth ; I wonder if what it means is that you broke some law, just to come back for the sake of—of that Harry ? " And by this time our author has, I think, left us in no doubt as to what law she had broken—the law that requires under penalty of deterioration of our whole personality that we should accept to the full the responsibilities that life throws upon us, that we should go on and not look back.

But Mary Rose's search is ended and she is set free. The voices call her again, and " the weary little ghost knows that her long day is done ". Trustingly, peacefully she steps out into the night of stars and vanishes. The play is ended.

Here I think Barrie means that, not as an individual, but as part of a much greater unit shall man ultimately find rest. That I believe is the conclusion to which many minds are tending these latter days. But that lies outside my present topic.

I am acutely conscious that I may have two very different points of view to encounter ; one that Barrie is too sentimental be be worth consideration ; the other that his work is too beautiful to analyse it thus. My reply to both such views is much the same—it is worth while to find out what the author really means if he can teach us something. You may ask whether he meant it consciously ; are you prepared to tell me whether Titian realized the tremendous psychological significance of his glowing harmonies of colour ? Well, let us agree that geniuses do not entirely comprehend the significance of their own work ; it makes us feel cleverer, at any rate, because we think we do. But I do feel that in *Dear Brutus* and *Mary Rose* Barrie has found himself more fully than ever before, and knew what he meant.

I am supported in that view by his posthumously

published autobiography, *The Greenwood Hat*, wherein he told us that he was naturally left-handed, but learned to write with his right, until he contracted writer's cramp and had to re-educate his left hand. He went on to say: " I write things with the left or, to put the matter I think more correctly, it writes things with me that the right would have expressed more humanely. I never, so far as I can remember, wrote uncomfortable tales like *Dear Brutus* and *Mary Rose* till I crossed over to my other hand. I could not have written these as they are with my right hand any more than I could have written *Quality Street* with my left." Evidently his readers are much indebted to his writer's cramp ! Now some authorities regard this disability as a revolt of the unconscious. I saw a patient whose cramp first developed over writing cheques for his wife, a process he had good cause to dislike cordially. Barrie's right hand perhaps refused to go on " writing with him " things which were plastered over with a deliberate sentimentality and not true to his deeper self. Being congenitally left-handed he acquired the power of writing that way late in life with comparative ease, and a rich outpouring from the unconscious was released through the more primitive route.

For to me the chief attraction of Barrie's work is the frequent employment of primitive imagery, of which I have already given examples. I find another in the closing scene of Peter Pan when he places the Wendy House on the tree-tops in Kensington Gardens, for Dr. Bosanquet suggests that the tendency of boys at a certain age to build shelters in trees is a reversion to the arboreal state of men.

It is a tremendously important fact that every one of us has to resume and repeat in nine short months the whole history of life on the earth, from its very inception as a single protoplasmic cell. No wonder if after this breathless flight we arrive a little puzzled by our environment. Making lungs and a heart—that's easy, it has been done so many times, though even that is occasionally bungled. But when it comes to harmonizing ourselves with our environment, that's all so new. The attempt hasn't been made 400 times in succession yet. Put 400 " greats " on to your grandfather and you find him squatting in a cave, gnawing rhinoceros' bones. And then the environment keeps changing too. It's a relatively uncharted sea—and, of course, we are too proud to learn from the mistakes our predecessors made. Evolution is a slow process, and has only been recognized as a fact for a little over sixty years. Our grandfathers thought the world was created in 4004 B.C.— it takes a little time to realize all that is implied by the much vaster outlook that evolution teaches us.

Physical infantilism we have clearly recognized for years, and psychological infantilism calls for equal recognition. When one realizes the difficulties that beset growing up, it is surprising that we accomplish it physically and psychologically as well as we do. Failure to do so adequately lies at the root of most psycho-neuroses.

Swinburne, whom I quoted just now, seems to me an excellent instance of the difficulty of growing up, which is in contrast to that of Barrie because there was a physical cause. Listen to this description of the poet's appearance while he was at Oxford. " The forehead startlingly white and large under its masses of red hair, squares well with the broad brows and the straight and level eyes below. . . . But the little loose lower lip, the tiny receding chin below suddenly mar the beauty and the seriousness of the whole, giving it at once a touch of the leonine and the elfin, a touch not so much of the grotesque as of the acutely disturbing."

This description implies that the narrow base of Swinburne's skull imprisoned his pituitary gland, preventing it, and therefore him, from growing physically, and then shut in his active brain till it was limited to turning over and over again the stock of ideas it had accumulated early in life. And I think we can see in the following quotations from Harold Nicolson the perennial struggle between the massive brain above and the cruel, cramping prison of that skull base below.

" From the age of nine his ambition centred upon the army. On leaving Eton he made a determined effort to enter the Dragoons. The proposal . . . was clearly grotesque, but the disappointment [at the refusal] was as galling as it was permanent. . . . This curious obsession, this pathetic virility complex, is significant not only of Swinburne's persistent inability to realize with any actuality either himself or his surroundings, but also of his continual struggle against the incomplete physical development which separated him from the normal male."

" Swinburne's emotional receptivity began to ossify in his twenty-first year. The experiences which he had by then absorbed became his future attitudes ; all subsequent experiences were little more than superficial acceptances. . . ."

" The ' internal centre ' of Swinburne was, I am convinced, composed of two dominant and conflicting impulses, namely the impulse towards revolt and the impulse towards submission.

" Swinburne quivers solitary, tremulous, aloof—as some lone seagull above the waves. . . . It was not, however, merely the aloofness of a sea-bird which appealed so insistently to his imagination, it was predominantly, perhaps, the quality of liberation and escape. . . . And, meanwhile, he strained and fluttered vehemently against the bars. This hatred of imprisonment, this obsession almost of claustrophobia, can be traced throughout the course of his otherwise acquiescent childhood ; the mutinous moods of his last year at Eton ; the hysterical outbursts at Balliol. His early manhood was but a constant defiance of circumstances, a hectic search after new worlds to startle or defy. Again and again we find him tilting wildly at windmills, attacking conventions which had already ceased to exist. Nor was this to him of any consequence, for what he loved was revolt only for the sake of revolt. And then in the end came Watts-Dunton and Putney, and the fine fire of mutiny was dimmed to a little lambent flame of wistfulness.

" As a counterpart to this volcanic violence there stands his curious docility ; an apparent causeless revolt matched by an apparently causeless submission ; for submission also he loved as an absolute quality, and for its own sake alone. Thus whereas Swinburne was always escaping he never ran away."

The province of medicine is co-terminous with life. Nothing that throws light on life is alien from the subject to which we have to devote our very existence. Psychology places a new weapon in our hands, a new means of combating suffering. It refuses to accept the theory that man is merely a test-tube in which certain chemical reactions occur. To understand all the affirmations it makes will transcend the lifetime of anyone here present. But the life of an institution like this is not limited to three score years and ten. Some of us remain here till our heads are as grey as the walls of this old Hospital, and our arteries grow almost as hard. But you represent the new life that is always pouring in, and it is for you to carry on the task, sustained by a vision of medicine as it is yet to be.

ROBERT BRIDGES: THE POET OF EVOLUTION[1]

When I received your Secretary's welcome invitation to address you, I had recently come from Stockholm, and as before, had been stirred by the presence of a new inspiration and a new art. It made me wonder, is Europe to be revivified again from the North as it was a thousand years ago by the Norsemen? For that Europe is mortally sick and in urgent need of transfusion who can doubt? At the time I was re-reading Robert Bridges's *Testament of Beauty*, and speculating on the next phase of evolution; your invitation arriving at that moment, some of those speculations were precipitated in a more concrete form. It seemed to me appropriate that I should, in this hall of all places, try to do honour to a great son of St. Bartholomew's—Robert Bridges the poet of emergent evolution.

Biology and the physics of the infinitely great and the infinitely little have in this century become the most poetic of all studies But I have felt for some years that before biology could appeal to the imagination, it needed a poet. The old saw has it " I care not who makes the nation's laws, if I can make its songs ". Biology has its laws; it needed its singer and found one in Robert Bridges. If I were to venture to suggest that in his time Tennyson had sung of evolution, I should fear the scathing criticism of a youthful audience. As well might I praise Mendelssohn. In these respects I bow to the judgment of my juniors and pass on.

What manner of man was Robert Bridges? I never met him. My impressions of him at Bart's were chiefly

[1] Being the Inaugural Address delivered before the Abernethian Society, St. Bartholomew's Hospital, on 3rd November, 1931.

derived from Sir Norman Moore, who stimulated me when I was secretary of this Society to ask him to address it. The reply came that he had nothing to offer which was worthy of our acceptance, which perhaps was not meant to be so complimentary as it sounds. But as people subsequently found when he was Poet Laureate, Bridges would never perform to order. He would not even contribute a poem to our Octocentenary celebrations. The wind bloweth where it listeth.

I will merely stress a few salient points in Bridges's life. He was born on 23rd October, 1844, and at the age of ten went to Eton. There he subsequently formed a warm friendship with a kinsman who was four years his junior and his fag, Digby Dolben. Dolben was accidentally drowned at the age of 19, but not before he had shown himself a poet of rare promise. These poems were, however, not published until 1911, when Bridges edited them and wrote a memoir of the author, which is of great value as revealing much of his own literary development as a boy. He shows that Dolben's approach to poetry was emotional, while his own was intellectual. Thus he says that Dolben " would never have written on a subject which did not deeply move him, nor would he attend to poetry unless it expressed his own emotion. . . . What had led me to poetry was the inexhaustible satisfaction of form, the magic of speech. . . . My own boyish muse was being silenced by my reading of the great poets. . . . My last serious poem at school was a sentimental imitation of Spenser. . . . I was abhorrent towards Ruskin . . . and well as I loved some of Tennyson's early lyrics and had them by heart, yet when I heard *The Idylls of the King* praised as if they were the final attainment of all poetry, then I drew into my shell, contented to think that I might be too stupid to understand." In these respects he anticipated modern taste, and I believe that *The Idylls of the King* is the chief cause of the present depreciation of Tennyson. King Arthur in the guise of the Prince Consort has been too much for us and has blinded a good many to Tennyson's real achievements. But to proceed, Bridges says : " As for Browning I had no leanings towards him. . . . In reading Shakespeare . . . my imperfect understanding hindered neither my enjoyment nor admiration. I also studied Milton and carried Keats in my pocket . . . [but] Milton was to Dolben as Luther to a papist . . . I had been dazed by the magnificence of the first book of *Paradise Lost* and gave no more heed to its theology then than I do now."

Both Bridges and Dolben were beginning to question the faith in which they had been brought up, but as Dolben tended more and more to Rome and Bridges more to science, their sympathies were drifting apart, and they had not corresponded for eight months before Dolben's death. But there can be little doubt that Dolben profoundly influenced Bridges in many ways, as any reader of this memoir can see.

Bridges went to Corpus Christi College, Oxford, in 1863, where he stroked his College Eight, but only obtained a second class in " Greats ". After leaving Oxford, he travelled for four years in Egypt, Syria, and Germany before entering St. Bartholomew's Hospital in 1871, at the age of 27, and therefore considerably older than the ordinary student. Although he published his first book of *Shorter Poems* as a third year student, he appears to have hidden his light from his fellows in those early days, for Dr. Winter, of Wolverhampton, who qualified from this hospital more than fifty years ago wrote to me as follows :—

" Years long ago that poets say were golden—
Perhaps they lay the gilding on themselves—

" I used to walk in Regent's Park with Robert Bridges. From his long cloak and soft hat, he looked like a tenor, but I had no idea that he was a poet, when he encouraged me to spout Keats and Shelley to him." In 1876, however, he published a Latin poem on the hospital and its teachers, several of whom were my own teachers nearly twenty years later. While he was House Physician he wrote a paper on the treatment of rheumatic fever by splints, which serves to remind us of the fearful sufferings endured by patients with this disease before salicylates were introduced. But it was when he became Casualty Physician that his most considerable contribution to medical literature was made. His " Account of the Casualty Department " published in vol. xiv of the *Hospital Reports* for 1878, has become a classic. This paper secured two things—one, that improvements were gradually made after his caustic exposure of the system— the other, that he was never given another appointment in the hospital. The powers that be do not appreciate irony, and youthful reformers still find it advisable to curb their tongues and pens. Unfortunately it still remains true that as long as the charitable public are influenced by the advertisement of the enormous numbers of patients treated at hospitals, no serious attempt will be made to deal with hospital abuse, but as Bridges said : " Since the days of David, the pride of numbers has never received such crushing rebuke as they have meted out to hospital statistics." In a year he saw 30,940 patients, an average of 1·28 minutes being given to each. That this was the usual state of affairs is corroborated by another paper on the Casualty Department in the same volume of the *Reports* by Dr. Norman Moore, as he then was. Bridges goes on to say : " If a casualty physician were to complain of the number of cases he has to see, he would probably be told that he is not supposed to attend to them or prescribe for them very much ; that the surgery is the filter of the hospital, or that he himself is the filter. It is in vain to point out that the filtering is of necessity a process slow in proportion to its efficacy, while the quick filtering of patients is almost unintelligible. Making bricks without straw cannot be compared to it ; that is done every day, but filtering quickly is a contradiction in terms. And yet filter he must, and filter quickly, too ; and be prepared to hear his quick filtrate shamefully ill-spoken of in the wards and in the outpatients' rooms."

However many patients pass through the Casualty Department to-day, and whatever the difficulties, we have a much larger staff to cope with them. In those days on the medical side there were only the junior assistant physician and three casualty physicians—no junior house physicians existed then. And those of us who remember and who worked in the old surgery realize the enormously better conditions under which the work is done to-day. Some of the surgical firms in my days as student, resident, and casualty physician merely worked behind screens of American cloth. As this state of affairs continued until 1906 when a temporary building was erected on the Christ's Hospital site, it will be observed that reforms were not carried out with undue haste. It is really impossible to do justice to this paper of Bridges by quoting extracts —it must be read in its entirety. In his calculations as to the cost of the different medicines, however, he touches a lighter vein. A bottle of the quassia and iron mixture, generally then called by the patients the " Queen Anne " mixture, because they mistook the taste of quassia for quinine, cost $1\frac{1}{8}d.$, while a certain famous mixture only cost 0·85286$d.$ per patient of which the greatest part was spent on the sweet colouring matter. But I would suggest that the rosy glow thus imparted to the mixture is of no slight therapeutic value. Bridges's experience did not lead him to subscribe to the view that " idleness is the casualty patient's excuse for coming to the hospital, and an hereditary taste for anything out of a bottle the unconscious motive of their seeking medicine." But he did not regard the existence of this type as wholly a myth, for he said : " It was only the other day that one of our patients when asked what was the matter with him replied : ' Well, sir, I don't know that there is anything the matter with me, but as I was passing the Hospital, I thought I would just step in and have a dose of medicine.' I should have been sorry to have drunk the dose that was prepared for him."

The admirable obituary notice of Bridges in the St. Bartholomew's Hospital *Journal* rightly says of medical poets that it must be confessed that though many of them may have been good doctors, few of them were good poets and that in the nineteenth century only three names, indeed, emerge above the level of mediocrity— Beddoe, Keats, and Bridges—and of these the greatest did not carry his medical studies beyond their early stages. Bridges is therefore to be regarded as the chief representative of the medical profession in this branch of the creative art during the last hundred years. I might add that in his early years Bridges took his profession seriously. He became Assistant Physician to the Great Ormond Street Hospital for Sick Children and the Great Northern Hospital. But he told Sir Norman Moore that he did not seek further promotion at Barts. because he realized that in those days the only avenue to the Staff was through the post-mortem room. In 1881 he had pneumonia and retired from the practice of medicine ; it has been stated that he always intended to retire at 40 and to devote himself to literature, but that he was convinced that he would be a better poet if he learned and practised some profession which brought him into active contact with human life and particularly with the investigations and achievements of natural science. We are therefore justified in concluding that he wished his poetry to express the philosophy of life he acquired from natural science in general and from medicine in particular. For this reason alone my title this evening would be amply justified.

For twenty years he resided at Yattendon, where his literary output was considerable, not only in poetry, but in criticism and on the subject of the spelling and pronunciation of English. He was one of the founders of the Society for Pure English. The last twenty-five years of his life were spent at Boar's Hill, Oxford, which seems likely to become the traditional home of the laureate muse.

In 1900 the Royal College of Physicians honoured themselves by electing him to the Fellowship. His appointment as Poet Laureate in 1913 was rather unexpected, as he had studiously avoided publicity and popularity. The early history of the Laureateship is somewhat vague. The first genuine official laureate was Bernard Andreas, who came over with Henry VII in 1485. Then the office appears to have been vacant until Dryden was appointed in 1663. Dryden was deposed in favour of Shadwell at the Revolution in 1688. Then followed a long line of indifferent versifiers who punctually produced Birthday and New Year Odes to be set to music and sung by the children of the Chapel Royal, Savoy. But when Southey was appointed in 1813 he resisted this custom, and since then the Laureate has had no set duties. Wordsworth followed Southey in 1843. Tennyson who succeeded Wordsworth in 1850 managed to combine his official duties and poetry with greater success than his predecessors, but on his death there was a widespread feeling that the post was an anachronism and might be allowed to lapse. Unfortunately, when Lord Salisbury became Prime Minister again in 1895 he reverted to the practice of the eighteenth century and advised the appointment of Alfred Austin. The successive appointments of Bridges in 1913 and Masefield in 1930 have helped to restore the prestige to the Laureateship which was so lamentably lost by that apparently cynical procedure. Bridges strictly adhered to Southey's refusal to write to order, despite the nagging of certain newspapers, to which he replied tersely and col.o-quially.

On his eightieth birthday his friends and admirers, remembering his life-long interest in music, presented him with a clavichord made by Arnold Dolmetsch. I like to think of that strikingly handsome old man, in a beautiful setting, playing his beloved Bach on a well tempered clavichord in the evening of his days. He achieved something that Milton only aspired to—for he was himself a true poem. But he was singularly favoured by fortune, though he suffered one " mortal distress " as he himself calls it, in the death of his daughter Margaret. Characteristically he tells us how he took refuge in beauty in that time of trial.

His greatest work, which was published in 1929, on his eighty-fifth birthday contains the choicest essence of his life-long thought. Nowell Smith tells us that while he was engaged upon it, he used to speak of it as his D.H.N. (i.e. " De Hominum Natura ") with allusion to the famous philosophical poem of Lucretius, " De Rerum Natura." He could not find a title to his mind until one day he suddenly announced that he had got it—the name was to be " The Testament of Beauty ". Nowell Smith goes on to say : " There have been many other versified treatises on the nature of things, on God, on Man, on the Soul, on the Universe. But nobody reads them either for their poetry or their philosophy, the reason being not that their authors were feeble philosophers, which they often were not, but that they were not real poets. Pope was not a real philosopher, but he was a real poet. Lucretius was both ; Robert Bridges was both. . . . ' The Testament of Beauty ' is a philosophical poem which bases itself upon the theory of Evolution popularly associated with the name of Darwin, as definitely as the ' De Rerum Natura ' based itself upon the atomic theory of Democritus as developed by Epicurus. . . . There has been an age-long antagonism between morals and religion, on the one hand, and art and poetry on the other. The earlier phase of the Renaissance was an attempted harmony ; but it was soon broken up. The High Renaissance stands over against the Reformation as Art without conscience against Morality without taste. It is only as a result of the liberating force of the scientific spirit that Beauty has begun to vindicate its place in the trinity of the absolute values. Thus it has come about that ' The Testament of Beauty ' is the first great didactic poem of æsthetic philosophy, and as such it seems likely to have an historic advantage over other long poems in an ever-increasing stream of literature."

A recent writer has said of Bridges that in spirit he was the most akin to the Elizabethans. " The songs of the Elizabethans, for all their spontaneity, spring to life already intricate and sophisticated in form ; as a flower opens, with its petals, the fanciful conceits of nature, already perfected and symmetrical. In such a union of spontaneous feeling with finished, ingenious craftsmanship Bridges is more fundamentally like the Elizabethans than in the particular rhythms and turn of phrase that he caught from them. . . . Because he was not deceived by the law of cause and effect, but knew how far astray it goes when it touches human feeling, his poems, even those which are fancifully written, give a special sense of reality, for they belong to a world in which things happen in the way we know."

Desmond MacCarthy says : "Unlike most poets his earlier poems have on the whole less emotion in them than his later ones. . . . He had from the first set his face against expressing black thoughts or pain. . . . Indeed he excluded them too resolutely. . . . But there was another sieve through which the intimations of the poetic impulse had to pass in his case, beside this reluctance to record black thoughts or pain. He was determined to illustrate only reveries which harmonize with the life of man as a social being, valuing only a temperate and rational beauty and selecting for poetic praise those things which cohere together in a happy and confident response to life as a whole. This implies his limitations." To which I would reply that these limitations were the almost necessary consequence of his sheltered life, but that within them, and because of his happy security from many of the anxieties that beset the ordinary man, he was able to achieve work of rare distinction. Not all great poetry is written in a garret. For as *The Times* said of him : "Both action and contemplation mixed in him with happy consequences to his generation and never let him grow old. . . . As time goes on, he will be recognized not only as a true English poet, but as one of those poets which nations, or circumstances, produce only at rare intervals."

Of the technical construction of his poetry I forbear to speak, as of something outside my province. There is no need to be antagonized by his simplified spelling—the eye quickly adapts itself to that. The rough-hewn lines

seem dissonant at first to an ear attuned to the smooth
Tennysonian rhythms—just as modern sculpture is trying
to the eye accustomed to classical forms. But a modern
poet, who was always experimenting in rhythms, told
me that when he thought he had arrived at something
new, he found that Robert Bridges had been there before
him. Another writer has told me that the internal
rhymes in the poem are a sheer joy to him. On this side
he is a poet's poet, and the ordinary reader will remain
content with the depth and beauty of his thought. No
one could have written " The Testament of Beauty "
without a biological training and, I should feel nclined
to add, without medical knowledge. That a man of
over eighty should have written such a poem is in itself
sufficiently remarkable, but that he should have
assimilated recent work on astronomy, archæology,
physiology, and psychology and have welded them into
new forms of beauty is to me amazing.

I do not think that the philosophy of Robert Bridges
was ever more succinctly expressed by him than in the
Broadcast Lecture on Poetry, which he delivered on
28th February, 1929. He spoke through the mouth of an
imaginary poet, who was, however, really himself.

" Now, if you don't like my poet, that is not my fault.
But if, as I guess, some of you suspect that he is going to
be too fantastical for your taste, I would reassure you on
that point ; for though he was a bit of a Platonist, he was
something of a Materialist since, holding that all our
Ideas come to us through the animal senses, Reality
(or our notion of Truth) must (as he affirmed) appear in
external forms to our thought ; and we must see Man's
Life on this planet as a Material Evolution (as most of us
in these days have come to regard it). And that Evolution,
as we see it, is a Progress from lower to higher, from what
we call Material to Intellectual and Spiritual in successive
stages from the Physicist's Atom to the Mystic's Vision
of God.

" Now, as my poet went on to say, Man's mind, being
such a receiver of Eternal Ideas, would be complete and

perfect if it received all the Ideas, and such a human mind would be abso'utely in harmony and at one with the Universe, as he is a part of it. But his animal condition is imperfect, and each man can receive only some of the Ideas, and those but imperfectly. . . .

" Such imperfection must be in all men's minds, and our minds differ according to the ideas by which each man is possessed. . . ."

This passage might indeed serve as a preface to his " Testament of Beauty ". The poem itself is in four books. The first consists of a beautiful introduction, wherein the poet describes how late in his long life-journey, having climbed to where the path was narrowing and the company few, he gained a new hill-top vision and realized the unity of all life, which forms a little oasis in Nature's desert. He saw in all existence, four stages—atomic, organic, sensuous, self-conscient. Our task is first to learn *what* is, before we attempt to inquire *why* things are as they are. We cannot sit in judgment on Nature, since we ourselves form a part of it. We can only reach an appreciation of beauty through our senses ; beasts have keener senses than ours, but it is reason that enables us while enjoying our senses to give them spiritual significance. This spiritual elation and response to Nature is Man's generic work. Man's mind, Nature's own mirror, cannot be isolated from her other works, but his conscious reason forms but a small part of his whole mind. Ask what is reasonable and one finds that time and clime conform mind more than body to their environment. Thus what seemed reasonable to St. Thomas Aquinas seems strange and unpalatable to him. Mere reason is not enough.

The mind of Hellas blossomed with a wondrous flower such as never since appeared among men. But gradually physical prowess outpaced spiritual combat with the Greeks ; they sought Empire and in consequence were molten into the great stiffening alloy of Rome. This introduction closes with a beautiful passage showing how the coming of Christ brought new spiritual values into the world. Thus we can pass from the sensuous, through the rational, to the spiritual in our evolution.

The Second Book opens with his main theme based on the vision of Socrates who saw the Spirit of Man as a chariot drawn by two winged horses. The Charioteer is Reason, but unlike Socrates he does not take one horse to represent good and the other evil ; he names them Selfhood and Breed. To each of these a Book is devoted, while the fourth is entitled Ethick, wherein he deals with the development of Reason's control over the instinctive impulses for the benefit of the community. Thus he agrees with Dupré's classification of impulses as those of self-preservation, concerned with the life of the individual, self-reproduction, concerned with the life of the species, and the gregarious habit, concerned with the life of the community. Each of these themes is taken up in turn, and with a wealth of imagery made to illustrate the principle of emergent evolution towards higher things. It is impossible to give any adequate abstract of all this without injury to the argument. I would, however, call special attention to his account of the evolution of maternal love and of the first dawning of ethical principle in which he imagines the nest-building bird making " conscient passage from the *must* to the *ought* ". Thus in man physical instincts were shapen to moral ends, or actually opposed by placing beside *ought* the equivalent *ought nots*.

The whole poem is a wonderful exposition of the direction in which I find a good many minds are set to-day—a sense, however shadowy, of what the next phase of evolution will be.

In all matters of this kind, the personal equation of the interpreter must influence his interpretation. The human mind cannot photograph, though it may portray. The angle of vision must differ with the individual. Which is only a paraphrase of what I quoted from our author. Will you therefore forgive the interpolation of a personal note by which I can perhaps make clearer my own point of view.

When I was only three weeks old the second Empire

met its debacle at Sedan and Napoleon III fled to England. When I was five weeks old Garibaldi entered Rome and overthrew the temporal power of the Pope. When I was but a few months old the German Empire was proclaimed at Versailles. I do not claim that I can remember any of these stirring events, but the effect of them on my seniors was to convince them, how erroneously we now know, that the frontiers of Europe were set for all time and that the days of war between the Great Powers were over. This sense of stability was communicated from the environment to the growing mind of the child. Some allowance must doubtless be made for the sense of time in a child, when the interval between one birthday and the next seems a whole epoch. But when all such allowance is made, it must be admitted, I think, that the seventies of the last century were extraordinarily stable and static. Early impressions such as these coloured the whole mentality of the men who had reached middle age when war broke out in August, 1914. As J. M. Keynes says, they regarded the then existing state of affairs as normal, certain, and permanent, except in the direction of further improvement, and any deviation from it as aberrant, scandalous, and avoidable.

In the eighties there was a stir of the æsthetic movement in art, and socially the almost sudden realization that industrialism had brought about conditions which must be remedied. Walter Besant's novels, *All Sorts and Conditions of Men* and *The Children of Gibeon*, stimulated the popular imagination and the People's Palace in Mile End Road was the direct result. It still carries on useful work as a technical college. Toynbee Hall and various college settlements in East London sprang up. There was a pathetic belief that with good will and mutual understanding a social millennium would arrive about 1930 ! Well, 1930 has come and gone and the social millennium seems much further off than it did fifty years ago. But no age has less reason to be ashamed of its dreams than the eighties of last century.

With the nineties a note of doubt and cynicism begins

to make itself heard. "Fin de Siècle" becomes the fashionable phrase. In the literary world the mid-Victorian
giants are dethroned and the Yellow Book is the manual of
the elect. But though its contributors proudly proclaimed
themselves decadent, they really seem, in the retrospect,
to have developed a new, delicate, and sensitive form of
art. In science Weismann chilled the expectation of
evolutionary progress by his denial of the possibility of
the transmission of acquired characters. In politics the
earlier somewhat theatrical imperialism of Disraeli and
the literary imperialism of the eighties as reflected in
Seeley's *Expansion of England* and Froude's *Oceana*,
hardened into the more materialistic imperialism of
Joseph Chamberlain and of Rudyard Kipling in his less
inspired moments. It rose to its zenith at the Diamond
Jubilee and crashed miserably in the Boer War as the
century ended.

Of the early days of the twentieth century, C. F. G.
Masterman said that there was a race between a horizontal
and a vertical line of cleavage, i.e. a cleavage between
classes or between nations. Nationalism just won, with
the results we know. C. E. Montague, who went to war
in the spirit of a crusader, has described in his book
Disenchantment the effect of the War on his and, indeed, on
most men's minds. Bridges himself spoke of

"War fallen from savagery to fratricide
From a trumpeting vainglory to a crying shame."

Few would deny that the War brought disillusionment.
We may have, as a consequence, gained in charity, we
have certainly lost much in faith and hope. I remember
about 1920 Sir Arthur Shipley saying to me, in that key of
humorous exaggeration he affected : "I agree with
Anatole France, that the creation of the universe was an
intolerably rash act." I subsequently found that there was
more of Shipley than of France in that phrase.

Do you remember three cartoons drawn by Max
Beerbohm about that time, which are now in the
Fitzwilliam Museum at Cambridge ? The first is "The

Future as seen by the Eighteenth Century ", and shows a brightly apparelled dandy gazing through a spy-glass at an attenuated image of himself. The second, " The Future as seen by the Nineteenth Century," shows a smug, stout, spectacled manufacturer gazing with satisfaction at a greatly enlarged image of—himself. The last, " The Future as seen by the Twentieth Century," shows a shell-shocked young man, with a mourning band on his arm, gazing apprehensively at a dark cloud bearing a large query mark. But note the subtle optimism of the artist. The eighteenth century was wrong, the nineteenth century was wrong, and perhaps after all our gloomy prognostications may be wrong as well.

Some of the reasons for this loss of confidence are obvious, others are more deeply seated. Man's reaction to nature varies with the control which he feels he has over it. The savage always went in fear of his environment, but our attitude became gentler and more romantic. We are the freer to admire the majestic contours of the mountain and the sunset glow upon them because we can ascend them in funiculars to rest in comfort in a well-equipped hotel, or burrow under them in a wagon-lit or fly over them in an aeroplane. But even to civilized man in the eighteenth century they presented a different aspect—these contours interposed barriers between him and his destination, the fading of daylight meant discomfort, difficulty, and even danger. And so his attitude towards mountains was quite different from ours. Despite Ruskin, no one really admired mountains before the age of railways. How much more awe-inspiring to primitive man was " Nature red in tooth and claw " than to us. Generally speaking, we felt so safe that a tornado, an eruption, or an earthquake struck us as vaguely unseemly and, paradoxically, somewhat unnatural. We became out of sympathy with primitive man's incessant efforts to placate nature since we had so largely conquered her external manifestations. But now, as I pointed out in my Maudsley Lecture, man has become much less confident of the control which reason can exert over his instincts.

Though we are far from returning to the theory of geological catastrophes which was widely held a century ago, we have departed from the conception of evolution as a smoothly continuous process and regard it as more probably occurring in a series of jumps. Indeed, the Quantum theory in physics suggests that all movement is of this order. Mutations are constantly recurring little jumps, but such geological changes as the oncoming or passing away of a glacial epoch must inevitably have produced much greater jumps. The whole of historic time is but as one day of evolutionary time, but even so we might have anticipated that we could detect some changes in man's physical structure in process. Wilfred Trotter indeed thinks that evolution can still be seen at work in lightening the cranium, the temporal muscles, and the jaws of the modern European. But on the whole we seem to be passing through a stable epoch as far as physical structure is concerned. Nor is there any real evidence of mental evolution. It would take some courage to assert that we have better brains than the ancient Greeks.

It would seem as if the vertebrates had now reached a rather similar dilemma to that of the invertebrates, for if man's brain were to become any larger, the chances of his being born alive would be greatly reduced. The lightening of the non-nervous structures of the skull to allow of some further increase of brain tissue, to which Trotter alludes, may do something, but if we have to depend on an increasing size of brain for further evolution, the dilemma would soon become acute both for mother and child. Are we to look forward to a race of Cæsarean-born, or rather is not this dilemma to be solved as was the former, by the development of a new co-consciousness ? Inevitably further evolution can only be psychological.

Gerald Heard makes a striking use of the well known conception of the evolutionary process as a spiral ; he maintains that our increased insight and interest in primitive men to-day, is due to the fact that in the spiral path of our own evolution we are looking directly down, as it were, into their minds, much as from an aeroplane, we can see the outlines of sites so long lost as to be hardly a legend. The discovery of the outer circle at Stonehenge and of Roman camps by this means are familiar examples. On the other hand, the horizontal displacement of even one generation ago was so great that their attempt to view the primitive mind failed in spite of the higher altitude. The observers saw little but the distorted reflection of themselves. It is interesting that he should use the same illustration of their attitude to the past that Max Beerbohm used for their attitude to the future.

It is this spiral advance which causes us to become rapidly out of sympathy with our immediate predecessors, for here only the lateral displacement shows itself, and to find ourselves strangely in sympathy in some respects, though not in all, with certain past epochs. Thus we are in sympathetic accord with much of the Greek thought, but find the idea of slavery as an essential feature of a city state quite distasteful to us. Professor Gwatkin said of the Middle Ages, in whose clothes so much of our religion is actually still arrayed : " We shall never quite understand them. We possess their work, but we are of a different spirit." I would say that our last tie with them vanishes as soon as we accept the idea of evolution. On the other hand, we appreciate the Humanism of the Renaissance but reject their failure in Humanitarianism. It may well be that the future will reject as valueless charity our humanitarianism as soiling the stream of life by strenuous efforts to preserve mental defectives while not preventing their reproducing themselves. Yet though the barbarity of our legal system of a hundred years ago revolts us, there are things in our criminal code of to-day which, as Richard Hughes said recently, will make as frightful reading to future generations as the proceedings of the Inquisition do to us ; and should they find in some forgotten drawer a faded photograph of ourselves, of you or me, with the memory of that record fresh in their minds, they will search our features in horror and surprise.

Obviously then our humanitarian attitude is not completely logical or logically complete, yet we could no more revert to the Renaissance attitude towards such things than we could revert to cannibalism.

Bridges has a remarkable passage in the first book of the Testament pointing out the utter slavery of the bee, however much this may be travestied by man's sentimental approach to the subject. Such communities would be incompatible with human happiness. But individualism in its present form is not enough.

Just as the solar system has an infinitesimal replica in every atom, so what we call an individual is a hive of minuter individuals. We are merely landlords for life— some of our tenants go on. But just as we contain cells that are living their own lives, so we form part of a greater individual. H. S. Jennings in his book, *The Biological Basis of Human Nature*, uses a striking metaphor. " Taken together, the generations constitute a great web or network. This network extends indefinitely forward and backward in time. It is formed by innumerable strands, the genes, which pass continuously through the net, which interweave and at intervals are gathered into knots, that we call individuals. From the knots, the strands again issue, separate, interweave with other strands, and form new knots, individuals of a new generation. . . . Every knot, every individual, is a new combination of strands, diverse from the combination forming any others, but containing strands that have been part of many earlier individuals . . . and will later pass to others. Of your store of genes you may say, as Iago said of his purse, 'Twas mine, 'tis his, and has been slave to thousands."

We are impressed by the instinctive knowledge of animals, but is it more striking than the instinct of the dividing ovum, each division knowing, as it were, exactly what to do. As Bridges says :

" 'Tis a task
incomparable in complexity with whatso'er
the bees can boast : nor do the unshapely cells behave
with lesser show of will, nor of purpose or skill."

But as C. E. M. Joad says : " Man's power of apprehending the universe grows. At each stage of his development he knows only so much of the outside world as he
is capable of apprehending, representing his guesses to
himself under the guise of myth and legend. Hence arise
religion, literature, and presently science, which is the
latest form of man's guesses about the world.

" At each stage of this developing knowledge there are
attempts to construct a building for the mind out of the
materials which have been acquired, a shelter of absolute
truths within which men may protect themselves from
the impact of fresh knowledge. There have been numbers
of these ' settlements ', as Heard calls them, in the history
of the race—the Church, the Reformation, the French
Revolution, and now Communism. The architects of each
' settlement ' demand that it shall not be a resting place
but a goal. In effect they say to Man's inquiring mind,
' You have found out enough. Further search is impious,
or unnecessary, or foolish, or impossible.' And always the
developing mind of man driven forward by the urge of
life, refuses to rest in the settlement and presses forward
to fresh horizons."

The next demand of evolution is clear—how to give
scope for the individual as a real entity and yet for him to
form as much a part of a greater whole as the cells do of
his own body. Here is a task for the choicest minds, and
the last part of Bridges's Testament shows how it occupied
his, and how he felt that " our happiest earthly comrade-
ships hold a foretaste " of the power to " surmount
humanity in some super-humanity." A very distant
but not impossible goal, for we are still but 'prentice hands
in the art of social relation.

You may well feel that here is a ha'porth of Bridges's
bread to an intolerable deal of my own sack. But you would
hardly expect a synopsis of the poem. I have merely
tried to tell you something of the effect it has had on my
own thoughts. I am a happier man for reading it, and if
I have encouraged any of you to read this rich flowering
of the wisdom of a generous, cultivated mind for yourselves

my object is achieved. It brings a wealth of consolation and calm to a distraught age. At the first reading the brilliance of the imagery, the striking illustrations drawn from history, science, and art may conceal how closely knit is the thought. But the remedy is simple—read it again.

SIR WILLIAM OSLER [1]

I shall not readily forget my first meeting with Sir William Osler, so magnetic was the effect, as with a quick elastic step he came forward in greeting ; his deep-set eyes darkly shining beneath the fine brow. A remarkable face ; not the least so because of the curious olive colour of his skin, the tone and texture of which caused both difficulty and merriment when he sat to Sargent for his portrait. I knew he was a great physician, but when I met him I knew I was in the presence of a great man, and many others have told me how they, too, experienced this instantaneous attraction.

Osler was not famous in the popular sense of the word with the general public, but none the less, his is a pervading influence alive among us to-day, for his effect upon the teaching and progress of medicine was subtle, widespread, and profound alike in England, Canada, and the United States.

Sir Archibald Garrod who succeeded him at Oxford spoke of him as one of those " men of light and leading who, like the Pied Piper of Hamelin, pipe a tune which others cannot but follow. Human sympathy and unselfishness are their chief weapons. Behind them their colleagues fall into line and around them they gather a group of disciples. In any international gathering Osler would draw around him friends from many nations ; he did more than any of his contemporaries to promote the brotherhood of medicine. He was unwilling to listen to detraction : his power of turning the conversation away

[1] A Broadcast given in the series " I Knew a Man " on Friday, 29th November, 1935.

from such talk was celebrated." Either a word of praise or silence was his rule.

William Osler was born in Canada on 12th July, 1849, the eighth child of Cornish parents. That impish, puck-like humour which he never overcame, manifested itself early, for he was expelled from his first school and was actually sent to prison for three days from his second for smoking out the matron by setting fire to a mixture of molasses, pepper and mustard ! It is therefore perhaps as well that he did not persevere in his original intention of going into the Church like his father before him. His love of natural history led him from theology towards science and thence to medicine. It has been said that he would have achieved greatness in any career, but it is certain that in no other walk of life would he have found so much exercise for his many gifts or fulfilled himself and been so happy as in the practice of medicine. His intense sympathy, his genius for friendship with young and old, his capacity for teaching and organization—for all these medicine gave ample scope. The keynote to his character was struck in a remark he made to his students— "There are people in life and there are many of them whom you will have to help as long as they live. They will never be able to stand alone."

Success came to him early, for he became a Professor at McGill University, Montreal, when he was only twenty-five, and a Professor he remained for the whole of the rest of his life, occupying chairs successively in Canada, the United States, and at Oxford, though no one could have been more unlike the conventional idea of a Professor. Before he was thirty he also became Physician to the Montreal General Hospital, where he at once made sweeping changes. The wards were made bright and cheerful ; all unnecessary evidences of illness were swept away. Many are the stories told of his kindness. Like St. Martin he gave his cloak one night to a beggar, who in return bequeathed to " my good friend William Osler " his liver, hob-nailed by drink. Another time when on his way to an evening party, seeing a sick child in the street he took him up in his arms and carrying him till he could find a cab, had him admitted to his hospital. His anxiety to conceal his feelings sometimes led to misunderstanding, for when deeply moved he was apt to put his hands in his pockets, tilt up and down on his toes and hum softly. Once when reproved for his seeming levity in such circumstances, he replied : " I hum that I may not weep."

Apart from medicine and his home life, Osler's great loves were old books, children, and practical joking. The first book he ever bought was a Shakespeare, and in later life he was able to help to restore the copy of the first folio to the Bodleian Library at Oxford which had been parted with many years before. His next purchase was Sir Thomas Browne's *Religio Medici*, and he ultimately collected a copy of nearly every one of the fifty-five editions of that work. It exactly fitted his humour for he was a deeply religious man, and he said that the author's own example showed that the perfect life may be led in a very simple quiet way. His appetite for books, rare editions, finely printed, bound, and illustrated steadily increased the more he was able to satisfy it. Here is a characteristic incident. A friend was talking to him of some book when Osler rose from his chair and, unlocking a little cupboard by the fireside, drew out the book in question. " I keep these particular books locked up," he said, " I am so afraid I might steal them myself." He left his library of nearly 8,000 books, classified on an original plan, to McGill University where they are splendidly housed.

To children he was indeed the Pied Piper, and when he piped they needs must follow, dancing. To turn up at a nursery tea was one of his favourite relaxations, usually in character—sometimes tiger, sometimes bear, of graphic realism. To children he dashed off innumerable letters in the course of his crowded day, usually purporting to be the advice or adventure of his tabby cat, and these were signed—Katamont, King of Kats.

All this was well, but when he carried such methods beyond the nursery into ordinary life, misunderstandings were bound to arise, and they did. Sir James Barrie has told us that he gave the name of McConnachie to the unruly half of himself which led him into pranks. Osler called his unruly and worse half Egerton Y. Davis, who wrote and did things of which the saner half would not approve. His friends sometimes prayed for Egerton Y. Davis's decease, for his practical jokes were audacious and occasionally cruel, which was entirely out of keeping with the rest of his character. But the boy who smoked out the school matron survived in him to the end, for although Osler once said he had drowned Egerton in the Lachine Rapids, like Sherlock Holmes he returned to life. On one occasion at least he subsequently wished that half of him had kept silent. Probably to quite a number of people Osler is only known as the person who said that a man was too old at forty and ought to be peacefully chloroformed at sixty. As a matter of fact he was quoting from Anthony Trollope, and he did it to tease a colleague aged seventy-three who was sitting on the platform with him at the time. They exchanged friendly smiles at the jest, but it was seized upon by the reporters and given headline publicity. Osler disliked any reference to this incident, but it pursued him for the rest of his life. Some eight years later when an evening paper announced that he was to give the most unfortunately named Silliman Lectures, it added that he was the man who had made this pronouncement, and that he was now sixty-three. The paragraph was headed: "An appropriate appointment."

Osler's life falls naturally into three periods—in Canada, in the United States, and at Oxford. In Philadelphia his new methods brought a breath of fresh air to an institution which was then in some danger of becoming stagnant. His unconventional ways frightened them at first. In those bachelor days he was careless in his attire and not the well-groomed figure, carrying immaculate yellow gloves, he became after marriage. They were not accustomed to a consulting physician who rode in a street car, carrying his lunch in a black satchel. But they swiftly realized his worth. Thence he went to take part in the founding of a new medical school at Baltimore—the Johns Hopkins, where he had a free hand and made it, as it is to-day, so justly famous. He combined what he thought was best in the German and English methods of training medical students. The great feature in the English system is that from an early stage in his training the student is made to regard a certain number of the inmates of a hospital as *his* patients. He is responsible for them, under proper supervision, and he makes personal contacts with them as individual human beings. This is the finest possible way of impressing him with the idea that the patient who has the disease is as important as the disease that the patient has. If we can claim, as I believe we rightly can, that patients are humanely treated in hospitals it is due to insistence on this principle and Osler, while introducing more scientific methods, was emphatic in maintaining it. He was fortunate in his colleagues and they soon gathered an enthusiastic band of students, many of whom are now renowned. Out of his teaching there arose his great book, *The Principles and Practice of Medicine*, probably the last great text-book of medicine that will ever be written by one man, so vast has the subject now become. Two important outcomes of this book were that indirectly it created the Carnegie Institute, and interested Mr. Rockefeller in medical research so much that he gave endowments which have contributed incalculably to the benefit of humanity.

But the book led to a great increase in his happiness in another way. The future Mrs. Osler had refused to marry him till the book was published, and when it appeared he threw a copy into her lap and said : " There, take the darn thing ; now what are you going to do with the man ? " Considering the weight of the volume I hope this story is not literally true ! Anyhow, they were speedily and secretly married, and a very happy marriage it was. Many regarded his wife as at least as striking a character. Her practical capacity and her gifts as a hostess smoothed his path. She used to say that his philosophy was not for everyone. What a state of affairs it would have been had she not laid in a stock of food, for he would bring in half a dozen visitors for lunch without warning, or give week-end invitations and forget them. On one occasion he invited the members of a conference to a garden party, of which she learned by accident only two hours beforehand. Yes, it was a remarkably happy marriage, marred by one great grief, the death of their only son in the War.

By 1905 he was beginning to feel the strain of his manifold activities and when the Regius Professorship of Medicine at Oxford was offered him, his hesitation was resolved by his wife's cable " Accept at once ". He did, and again made a great success. He told a friend that he came over to England to get educated and to live within an hour or so of the British Museum. Just as his forwardly directed mind enabled him to make a new medical school at Baltimore, so his sense of the past made him revel in the charm of Oxford. It was a special delight that the Mastership of the Almshouses at Ewelme was attached to his Professorship. These cloistered buildings founded by Chaucer's granddaughter nearly 500 years ago appealed strongly to him, and so did the thirteen aged inmates whom he got to know so well, for he was the first Master within the memory of man to live among them. Rapidly he gained their affection, and when he died one old man said : " I'll see him soon ; he'd know me in a hundred, he would. God bless him."

That his house at Oxford should have been known as " The Open Arms " speaks for itself. It shows the same spirit that led him to found the Association of Physicians which stopped us from working in an isolation from one another that was by no means splendid. His geniality pervaded our meetings and his inspiration still remains among us. Once when a member resented Osler speaking of his " armchair speculations ", he took him by the arm and said : " My dear man, the best thing about these meetings is that anyone can say what he jolly well likes."

I well remember the gathering on his seventieth birthday soon after the War when Sir Clifford Allbutt, then in his eighty-fifth year, presented him with a memorial volume from friends and pupils, saying : "Through this clamour and destruction your voice, among all the voices in the serener air of faith and truth, has not failed, nor your labour for the sufferings of others grown weary." Osler could not trust himself to make an impromptu speech, so he read his reply ; a moving speech and when he tried to speak of his own loss he nearly broke down. For he never recovered from the death of his son, and soon afterwards a chill contracted in an attempt to return to his Oxford duties during the railway strike proved fatal. He might well have expected to live longer for his father lived to about ninety and his mother reached her centenary.

Despite all the honours which fell thick upon him in his later years, he remained unassuming and modest. " The profession has pushed me forward," he would say. " A few of my intimate friends really know the truth about me as I know it ! My brains, in good faith I say it, are of the most mediocre character. But what about those professorships you ask ? Just habit, a way of life, an out-come of the day's work." But great as his work was, the man was greater still. I am thankful that I had the privilege of knowing him. The gaiety that bubbled up spontaneously out of spiritual depths, his sanity and his courage, his intense sympathy, were among his many gifts to us. His presence and his touch brought comfort and healing. For his epitaph I would take the passage from Tennyson's Ulysses that he often applied to himself :

I am a part of all that I have met ;
Yet all experience is an arch wherethro'
Gleams that untravelled world whose margin fades
For ever and for ever when I move.

THE PSYCHOLOGY OF AUTHORSHIP [1]

It was a happy thought on the part of this Club to adopt the name of Osler, for he, of all men, had his eye directed towards the younger generation. I am told that this Oration may be on any subject in which Osler would have been interested—a wide field indeed, for he was interested in everything. Undoubtedly this topic comes within the four corners of the definition, passionately interested as he was in books.

In beginning with some aspects of authorship in the seventeenth century, I am actuated by two motives. The first is a personal one. When I was introduced to Osler he made a friendly allusion to me as the son of my father. For we both sprang from the same Puritan stock, and from his youth his mother had instilled in him an interest in John Bunyan, to whom my father was the sixth direct successor, and of whom he wrote the standard biography. The second is a more topical one : at the present moment there is a great revival of interest in seventeenth century literature. And there is good reason for this, for that age and the present have this in common : they are both ages of disillusionment.

No one, I fancy, would challenge the statement that this is an age of disillusionment. The enormous material advance of the nineteenth century begat an invincible belief in the Law of Progress, and in its latter half Manchester Liberalism and the doctrine of " *laisser-faire* " drew fresh sustenance from Darwinism after a preliminary revolt from such unaccustomed food. The struggle for existence and the survival of the fittest

[1] The Annual Oration delivered before the Osler Club on 12th July, 1933.

179

seemed to provide scientific sanction for its business methods. And then the skies changed; a preliminary rumble of thunder came from the Boer War; then the storm was upon us. Ruefully regarding the wreckage left by the passage of that tornado, doubtfully gazing around for fresh clouds which may burst upon our devoted heads, we realize indeed the shrewd winds of disillusionment.

In another way, and for somewhat different reasons, the seventeenth century was an age of disillusionment, which had started before the Civil War. It therefore interests us to see how our ancestors comported themselves after the excitements of the Elizabethan age. Man's impulse to classify perhaps tends to make him lay undue emphasis on the cleavage between one century and another, for our calendar is purely artificial in that respect. Yet who can doubt that with each of the two queens, Elizabeth and Victoria, an epoch also died?

On its intellectual and artistic side what a marvellous flowering was the Renaissance! We may attribute much to the new writings, that is to say printing, the new learning which was the old learning come to life again, and the new world across the Atlantic. All of these seemed to stimulate man's imagination in a way that had not happened since the Greeks rebuilt Athens after defeating the Persians. Yet its inner essence remains as mysterious as the springing of youth into adolescence. Of the Renaissance the late Sir Walter Raleigh, whose name and spirit alike are reminiscent of that time, wrote thus:

"That great movement of the mind of man brought with it the exhilaration of an untried freedom and the zest of unlimited experiment; but it took the human soul from its station in a balanced and rounded scheme of things, to deliver it over to every kind of danger and excess. . . . From his servant's estate in the great polity [of Catholic theology], man was released by the Renaissance, and became his own master in chaos, free to design and build and inhabit for himself. The enormous nature of the task, which after three centuries is still hardly begun, did not at first oppress him ; he was like a child out of school, trying his strength and resource in all kinds of fantastic and extravagant attempts."

If danger and excess, fantastic and extravagant attempts are to be put on the debit side, we may fairly put it on the credit side of the Renaissance that free inquiry was no longer stifled. It is an intriguing thought that if the attitude of the Middle Ages to scientific research still held, Lord Rutherford, Sir J. J. Thomson, and Marconi would certainly have languished in prison, if indeed they had not been burnt at the stake.

Gerald Heard, in his thought-provoking book, *The Ascent of Humanity*, expresses his point of view somewhat as follows : The Renaissance stated its problem and gave its solution, that man is an individual, and that he is free to take his satisfaction from Nature and the community. Up to the close of the sixteenth century the most active spirits had not got beyond that simplicity. This, under the thin disguise of a formal assent to religious *clichés* was still Bacon's attitude. Machiavelli's *The Prince* is fundamentally the product of a simple mind. It is not subtle ; it is only cynical ; the eternal commonplaces of virtue are merely reversed. If " Thou shalt love thy neighbour as thyself " does not make for success, then the opposite obviously must. But inevitably the Prince of Machiavelli is succeeded by Hamlet, Prince of Denmark. Bacon remains no more than the last great fruit of the Renaissance ; the highest development to which the speculative mind could attain if unaccompanied by a proportionate sensibility. He fulfilled the middle rôle between Machiavelli and Shakespeare. The theme that individuality, however intellectually endowed, is not enough, the recognition of a rudiment of feeling breaking through the surface of the self-contained mind is the fundamental obsession of Shakespeare. He cannot escape from the fatal irresolution which he discovers developing in his own consciousness and among his contemporaries.

The age had been one of almost frantic activity. The country of which he was a native had had every stimulant ; wild adventure in the ends of the earth, threats of destruction from abroad, constant plots within. Now it was beginning to sober down.

Whether Shakespeare was a syndicate or an individual, whether he was Edward de Vere, 17th Earl of Oxford, or not, in my opinion he certainly was not Bacon. And my principal reason for being so dogmatic is the kind of evidence I have adduced from Gerald Heard. Intellectually, at any rate, they were not really contemporaries. A gulf yawns between them ; a new sensibility has been born. Unlike Dante, who was always a judge, Shakespeare was a recorder and commentator.

In the drawing-room of the Master's Lodge at Trinity College, Cambridge, hangs a portrait of Bacon sufficiently sinister to make the onlooker uncomfortable. Yet I am informed that it is less sinister than the original one in the possession of his family which, when copied, has actually been altered, so evil is its expression. An interesting sidelight on his character !

The greatest proof of Shakespeare's genius to me is that each century has found something new in him. Regarded by certain of his contemporaries with something " this side idolatry ", to the seventeenth century he was fancy's child, warbling his native wood notes wild, and to the eighteenth century a master of rhetoric. Then the early nineteenth century found something unsuspected before or since, for Coleridge took him as a final and complete exponent of morals. He even went so far as to say that any characteristic not described by Shakespeare was not an important ingredient of human nature. Unfortunately for his thesis, he illustrated it by saying Shakespeare never described avarice, which was therefore not a fundamental human characteristic. True, Shylock was actuated more by revenge than by avarice, but Coleridge's idea seems to have been to make Shakespeare a Bible of human conduct. A curious conception of a man who had to write plays that would literally beat cockfighting if he was to attract audiences to his Bankside theatre from the neighbouring sports ! The Victorian age commended Shakespeare for his intelligent anticipation of the Victorian young lady, while ours finds in him an exponent of those psychological problems by which we are obsessed.

Then there is Pearsall Smith's view : " Once and once only in the history of a people, there comes a divine moment when its speech seems to those who write it a new-found wonder ; when its words are fresh with the dew of the morning upon them, when its language is in a plastic state, unstereotyped, unhackneyed, unexploited ; and it is at this moment that the one supreme poet appears ; for no form of language seems rich enough to provide material for more than one single poet of this rank.

" Such a supreme poet Shakespeare became ; in the great linguistic ferment of the 1590's he made himself the great lord of language, the most articulate of human beings."

Not that this expresses all of Shakespeare's magic. Like Lyly, he started as a euphuist, but he became much more. There is, by the way, the same sense of joyous discovery of a new language in the writings of Joseph Conrad, to whom also English was foreign and fresh.

Since writing this I have come across a cutting I made from *The Times Literary Supplement* some years ago. It serves to illustrate the point I have been trying to make :

" Now there seem to be, or to have been, two principal conditions under which poetry in the grand style has been written in the Christian era—conditions represented by Dante and Shakespeare respectively. One is the universal prevalence of a systematized religious faith offering symbols which express the mystery of human life, so that poetry can, without any sense of derogation or limitation, make itself ancillary to religion and ' justify the ways of God to man '. The other is the occurrence of a moment, naturally associated with the decline of a universal religious faith, when the individualistic view of life prevails, and the mystery of life finds expression in tragedy. These moments are not simply opposed to one other. They are phases in a historical movement. While Christianity was, consciously or unconsciously, the universal faith, tragedy was impossible; since Christianity obviously does not permit the tragic view of life. As Christianity weakens tragedy emerges. But manifestly the tragic view of life has no finality. As an individual and prophetic man, Shakespeare passed beyond tragedy. It would be a mistake to urge, as is sometimes urged, that he returned to Christianity; he rather passed from Christianity, through tragedy, to a reconciliation of a kind which, no doubt, was found in former days by chosen spirits in Christianity but is not uniquely Christian. Of all this movement in Shakespeare, Goethe, the first profound student of Shakespeare, was perfectly conscious."

But I am not embarking on the sea of Shakespearian criticism, which is bestrewn with so many wrecks. I am content to rejoice that the magic of his language increases for me with every year I live. Where he comes into my story to-day is that his later works marks the definite change of thought which happened because the Renaissance and the Reformation "had quickly fallen out of step". Things were proving not so simple after all. The counter-Reformation, too, was complicating things. Men began to cast up their losses and their gains. Hobbes, that forerunner of the materialistic rationalists, remarked in his *Leviathan* that since the Renaissance led to so much effusion of blood, "I think I may truly say that never was anything so dearly bought as these Western poets bought the learning of the Greek and Latin tongues." The political horizon was clouding too. All this is reflected in what Grierson has called the " cross currents in English literature of the seventeenth century", and of which he has written so illuminatingly.

The change is well illustrated by the difference between the earlier and the later writings of Donne, though the change from the extroversion of the sixteenth to the introversion of the seventeenth century is implicit in both. But I shall deal with the Anglican writers, such as Donne and Sir Thomas Browne, in another chapter. I prefer to illustrate my thesis from such Puritan writers as Milton and Bunyan, of whom I know rather more. Milton's case was complex, Bunyan's simple. I will take the simpler first.

John Bunyan's upbringing was of the humblest. There is a note in the diary kept by the Rector of the neighbouring parish about his father : " One Bonion of Elsto clyminge of Rookes neasts in the Bery wood ffound 3 Rookes in a nest, all white as milke and not a black fether on them." " And as we watch him, the surprise on his face becomes symbol and presage of a wider world's wonder than his, the wonder with which men find in the rude nest of his own tinker's cottage, a child of genius." Indeed, a white bird in the black rook's nest.

He lived sixty years and wrote sixty books. His prose was poetry and his poetry was prosy. His imaginative power was great, and Puritanism allowed of few outlets for it, except that of the religious allegory. It may be that the continued popularity of the *Pilgrim's Progress* is partly due to the fact that it was one of the few books which, in the stricter days of nonconformity, children were allowed to read on Sunday. Myself I have pored with delight over illustrated editions portraying Christian in deadly conflict with the laidly beast Apollyon, and followed the siege of Mansoul in *The Holy War* with quite another interest from that intended by the author. And then there was *Foxe's Book of Martyrs*, an early edition which had belonged to Bunyan himself—with illustrations of horrible tortures and burnings such as charm the sadistic strain to be found in most children. Yes, these were compensations which even that hymn, " A few more years shall roll," with its appalling threat of an " Eternal Sabbath Day ", could not quite obliterate. Augustine Birrell tells us how, in his early days, the title of *The Bible in Spain* allowed him to mitigate the Sabbath by revelling in George Borrow.

However, there is no doubt that the *Pilgrim's Progress* is a fine allegory written in fine English. But if we are to know Bunyan himself, we shall find the key in his *Grace Abounding to the Chief of Sinners*. The psychoneurotic note is struck at once. " The Chief of Sinners "—for the psychoneurotic must be the chief of *something*.

Bunyan was a sick soul in those earlier years. Literature owes much to the sick soul. If you want a skilful dissection of different types of the sick soul read William James's *Varieties of Religious Experience*. To the normal man such shuddering depths of despair and fear seem unreal, but they are real enough to the sufferer. Bunyan was obsessed with a sense of sin. When the history of thought in the nineteenth and twentieth centuries comes to be written, it will surely strike the writer that about seventy years ago the idea of sin began gradually to lose its hold over man's minds, and that to-day it has almost vanished for the great majority. And I should be surprised if that writer does not point out that this change is almost synchronous with the increasing hold of the idea of evolution. But obsessional states and anxiety neuroses continue among religious and irreligious alike. Religion does not cause them, nor, according to the histories which religious patients give me, does it cure them. Rather does the failure of religion to help them add to their torture, since they feel this must be due to some failure of faith on their own part. The falling and the lifting of the cloud seem equally mysterious in the present state of our knowledge.

Bunyan's anxiety neurosis shows the characteristic spread of a phobia. He tells us that he was fond of bell-ringing. Then he came to regard this as a sin. But he would still go and lean against the old doorway and look longingly while a neighbour pulled the bell-rope. Then he was afraid even to do this. How if the bells should fall ? How if even the steeple itself should come down ? About that very time a flash of lightning struck one of the village churches of Bedfordshire, and

" passing through the porch into the belfry, tripped up his heels that was tolling the bell, and struck him stark dead ". What if this should happen to him ? And so the phobia spread and spread.

Strange alternations of gloom and glory came over him. Sometimes he was visited by such visions of light and hope that he could have told his joy to the very crows of the field. He thought then that he should never forget the joy even in forty years' time. But alas ! in less than forty days the vision was all faded and gone : " Oh how happy now was every creature over I was ! for they stood and kept fast their station, but I was gone and lost." Then at last comes relief in his conversion, I hope you will not think me flippant if I suggest that this was a " conversion " in the Freudian sense of the term, for what really happened, as Grierson points out, was that " Bunyan's fear of the wrath to come made him afraid of nothing else ". I believe that is correct ; the fear of the unknown was less bearable than the fear of something which he thought he knew, and from which he felt he had the means of escape.

In allegory, too, one is tempted to think he found an escape. " He enjoyed writing and creating scenes and characters, drawing on his knowledge of the human heart and the human character, and also a little on those ' beastly romances ' which he had read in his youth. It is a partial emancipation. The main issue is never lost sight of. . . . Fear is the dominant emotion." It is an interesting fact that when he married a wife as poor as himself she brought with her two books, one of which was entitled *The Plain Man's Pathway to Heaven.* Herein he may well have found the germ of *The Pilgrim's Progress from the City of Destruction to the Celestial City.*

It has been pointed out that a Cluniac MS. of the thirteenth century, *Le Voyage d'une Ame,* contains too many of the incidents of *The Pilgrim's Progress* to be merely coincidence. As this MS. has only been recently translated into English it is impossible for Bunyan to have read it. He may, however, have heard its story at third or fourth hand.

Schirmer has emphasized the interesting fact that the Puritans, despite their condemnations of the drama and general disapproval of all secular literature that had only pastime for its end, were vital contributors by way of allegory to the rise of the novel, as a realistic picture of everyday life and character, and also as a vivid portrayal of the inner conflict of conscience and passion. I may remind you that Defoe was a dissenter, and therefore had stoutly to maintain that his romances were narratives of fact.

" But if the *Pilgrim's Progress* was a forerunner of the novel, *Grace Abounding* was the ancestor of Rousseau's *Confessions*, and James Joyce's *Portrait of the Artist as a Young Man*," says Schirmer. Strange adventures that link John Bunyan with James Joyce. But how different were their spiritual Odysseys !

Jack Lindsay in his recent biography ingeniously explains Bunyan's psychological state on strictly Freudian and Marxian lines. This has involved the device, so frequently employed by modern biographers, of assuming a knowledge of the inner thoughts of the man he portrays. While admitting that Bunyan gives no direct clue to any emotional recoil from his father's quick remarriage after his mother's death, he maintains that it shook him to the roots and was the origin of his religious distress. If we grant this, despite the absence of any direct evidence, we may perhaps accept his deduction: " Thus does the religious emotion feed on the sense of irresponsibility in the adult, parental world. . . . The baffled sense of social unity flows into the imagination of a Perfect Father." Certainly on those lines Bunyan can be fitted rather neatly into Freud's Procrustean bed. But surely Marx makes a strange and uneasy bedfellow. I am not so ready to agree that all Bunyan's spiritual distresses had a social-political origin—that he was a Marxian born out of due season. It is difficult to believe that all such distresses will cease to be in a classless society ; since man cannot live by bread alone this seems indeed a pathetic wish-fulfilment. The Marxian classless society is just as much an abstraction as Plato's Ideal Republic, More's Utopia, or Bunyan's Celestial City. Strange, is it not, that men hardly lose any time between rejecting one infallible bible and swearing allegiance to another?

The case of Milton was a more complex one as I have said, and one that is more illustrative of cross-currents.

I count it a gain that at school I was made to learn "L'Allegro," "Il Penseroso," "Lycidas," and the "Hymn on the Nativity" by heart. They are a storehouse of lovely imagery and have become for me an abiding possession. But I see now, as I did not then, that they also illuminate both the passionate and the Puritan sides of his nature, which waged perpetual warfare in him. His parents early made up their minds that he was destined for greatness. That, I believe, is not uncommon in parents! The result was, as Mark Pattison emphasized, that his early life was a long preparation for some great task which he felt was laid upon him, the exact nature of which it was not given to him at once to descry, though his natural aptitudes and inborn tastes pointed to a literary work, a great poem which should be an act of service to God and to his country. But his sheltered upbringing left him to some extent without armour for the contacts of a rough world. And Milton had to live through troublous times within and without. The way of idealists is hard, especially if they be also poets and egoists, and the "Milton who composed *Paradise Lost* was an angry and embittered man", says Grierson. "Much for this man, young, passionate, pure, would depend on the woman with whom he first fell seriously in love, and whom he should make his wife. That experience came to Milton simultaneously with the challenge that summoned him to leave the enchanted garden of culture and meditation, to take up his rôle in the world of action." The meeting of the Long Parliament in 1640 was for him the great awakening. "To the young man of 33 it seemed that a new age was beginning for the English people and the Christian church. . . . And then in the early summer of 1643 he made his

189

sudden journey into the country, 'nobody about him certainly knowing the reason, or that it was more than a journey of recreation,' and returned with Mary Powell as his wife. Of what led up to that marriage we know nothing and can only assume . . . that the susceptibility to passion of which his Latin poems give evidence, which his high ideals of purity and love, his religious temper and training, had kept in check took revenge upon him, and made him too hastily discover the ' well-beloved ' in a young girl of 17. The consequences were for him almost as disastrous as the very different marriage of Byron was for a very different poet. This first and fatal shock to a finely tempered and carefully nurtured and sheltered personality . . . coloured everything that he thought and wrote to the end of his life." You are to remember this point of view. His praise of chastity in " Comus " is so extreme as to seem to us to-day deliberately designed to defeat its own purpose, and was indeed recently so represented on the stage. But it was real to him. Here, indeed, was a crux. He was not disposed to accept the situation as irreparable. " If his marriage had gone wrong, the laws of marriage must be reconsidered," and that early summer had only deepened into August before he had published his *Doctrine and Discipline of Divorce*. " But among the most censorious critics of the doctrine of divorce are the Presbyterians, and they are the censors of the press. So Milton parts from his old friends." He writes his *Areopagitica*, a demand for the freedom of the press, pours contempt upon his opponents, and declares that new Presbyter is but old Priest writ large. His second marriage brought some promise of assuagement, but " his late espoused saint " died all too soon, as we know from one of his most beautiful sonnets.

We see that for Milton to feel a thing strongly it had to be part of his personal experience. This is seen even in *Paradise Lost*. The Homeric conflicts between God and Satan reflect the turmoil of his own soul. The idyllic scenes in the Garden of Eden represent the conquest of reason by romantic love, of which he had had bitter experience. But after that, when he is trying " to justify the ways of God to man " he becomes more didactic and far less interesting. I doubt if any of us remember much beyond the first four books. Seen in this light we can understand why Satan is made such an heroic figure— he represents Milton's own instinctive emotional self, struggling in the toils of social convention which bound him. Blake says that " Milton was of the Devil's party without knowing it ", though Blake's own illustrations to Job show more than a sneaking admiration for Satan. Landor is probably nearer the mark when he says that *Paradise Lost* is " not a justification of the ways of God to man as orthodoxy understands it, but an arraignment of orthodox conceptions of God and the Devil, a complete reversal of the apparent values of the poem ". Grierson sums up the situation when he says : " In Milton the creature imagination and the critical intellect did not work in such harmony with one another as they have in some other poets."

But that indeed is the crux for many writers, both of poetry and prose. Let me illustrate two different methods of resolving this conflict, both of which I regard as pathological.

Just after my first visit to Rome, some thirty-five years ago, I read a remarkable novel, *Hadrian the VIIth*, by Rolfe. In it an Englishman achieves the triple tiara and takes the title of Hadrian, because it is the same as that taken by Nicholas Breakspear, the only Englishman who ever became Pope. He renounces all claim to temporal power, aiming at solely a moral sovereignty over Europe. The people applaud, the Cardinals are scandalized, and Hadrian is killed by an assassin's bullet. As I read the story I became more and more convinced that the author had visualized himself as Pope. A few years ago I read an account of him by A. J. A. Symons which more than justified that idea. He took the title of Baron Corvo—where gained no one knows. He wrote several books, but this was the only one which attracted much attention, and he became more and more overbearing, quarrelsome, and impossible in every relationship of life. Those who knew him realized that he was always seeing himself as Pope, and as he was not treated as Pope he was fiercely resentful. He would begin a letter " Quite cretinous creature," and end another " bitterest execrations." It has been said that " to the world at large he seemed actuated by motiveless malice. . . . He saw the hand of an enemy in every misfortune ; and where he saw an enemy he struck." The fantastic image of himself that he constructed overflowed into real life ; the conflict became an external instead of an internal one. His condition was perilously near a psychosis, if it did not actually become one.

The second illustration is that of the author of *John Inglesant*. When I was entering my teens it happened that I came into a literary atmosphere which I enjoyed without comprehending. The people in it talked much of John Henry Shorthouse and his book *John Inglesant*. When I was thirteen his much-heralded second novel appeared—*The Little Schoolmaster Mark*. It was a complete and dismal failure. He proved to be emphatically a man of one book, but that book continued to have readers and admirers more than half a century after its first appearance when the author was regarded as a " minor prophet of things of mystical taste ".

Then in 1925 came a bombshell into literary circles when W. K. Fleming (afterwards Canon Fleming) published an article in the *Quarterly Review* entitled " Some Truths about John Inglesant ". He had discovered that this much-admired book was a regular mosaic of borrowed gems. His enlightenment came from reading in the *Diary of Thomas Ellwood* these words : " I was sitting all alone. . . . I felt a word sweetly arise in me, as if I heard a voice which said, Go and Prevail. And, Faith springing in my heart with the word, I immediately rose and went, nothing doubting ". The phrase had a familiar ring, and then Canon Fleming remembered that these were the words in *John Inglesant* used by Mr. Thorne in paying his addresses to May Collet of Little Gidding. Further search reaped a rich reward. The "liftings" were sometimes paragraphs, sometimes whole pages from many works. The extraordinary thing is that many extracts had been taken from books that are still read, and not merely from recondite sources. I might instance Evelyn's *Diary*, Hobbe's *Leviathan*, John Aubrey, Anthony à Wood, Burton's *Anatomy of Melancholy*. There were many others. Yet the book had been published forty-four years before this was detected. It suggests that we are not so well versed in seventeenth-century classics as we sometimes pretend to be.

Fleming's comment is that Shorthouse apparently drenched himself in literature contemporary to his tale of the seventeenth century, which he threaded together with his own really beautiful nineteenth-century English. " Shorthouse," he says, " probably looked on the book as a private labour of love never destined to see the light ; when persuaded by friends less versed than himself in the originals he found it impossible to tear out the borrowings without fatally disfiguring the whole." But this is hardly a complete explanation. Let us turn to the preface he wrote to the second edition and his defence of what he calls the philosophical romance, in the course of which he says : " Yes, it is only a Romance. It is only the ivory gates falling back at the fairy touch. It is only the leaden sky breaking for a moment above the bowed and weary head, revealing the fathomless Infinite through the gloom. It is only a Romance." Beautiful words, but not precisely informed with the humility of a conscious plagiarist.

Mr. Will Spens, the Master of my College, tells me that with full knowledge of these borrowings, he cannot believe that the mystery of *John Inglesant* is yet solved. He maintains that there is still much of Shorthouse in it. In particular he instances Inglesant's statement of the Catholic position in the Epilogue, which is only thus stated in one other work—and that a Russian book which has only recently been translated into English.

Soon after Fleming's revelations appeared I happened

to come across A. C. Benson's description of Shorthouse in *The Silent Isle*. It is important to remember that Benson died before these revelations were made :

" I have been reading the *Memoir of J. H. Shorthouse*, and it has been a great mystery to me. It is an essentially commonplace kind of life that is there revealed. He was a well-to-do manufacturer of vitriol, too, of all incongruous things. He belonged to a cultivated suburban circle, that soil where the dullest literary flowers grow and flourish. He lived in a villa with small grounds ; he went off to his business in the morning, and returned in the afternoon to a high tea. In the evening he wrote and read aloud. The only thing that made him different from other men was that he had the fear of epileptic attacks for ever hanging over him ; and, further, he was unfitted for society owing to a very painful and violent stammer. I saw him twice in my life ; remote impressions of people seen for a single evening are often highly inaccurate, but I will give them for what they are worth. On the first occasion I saw a small, sturdily-built man, with a big clerical sort of face with marked features, and as far as I can recollect, rather coppery in hue. There was a certain grotesqueness communicated to the face by large, thin, flyaway whiskers of the kind that used to be known as ' weepers ' or ' Dundrearies '. He had just then dawned upon the world as a celebrity. I had myself read and re-read and revelled in *John Inglesant*, and I was intensely curious to see him and worship him. But he was not a very worshipful man. He gave the impression of great courtesy and simplicity ; but his stammer was an obstacle to any sense of ease in his presence. I seem to recollect that instead of being brought up, as most stammerers are, by a consonant, it took the form with Shorthouse of repeating the word ' Too—too ' over and over again until the barrier was surmounted ; and in order to help himself out he pulled at his whiskers alternately, with a motion as though he were milking a cow. Some years after I saw him again ; he was then paler and more worn of aspect. He had discarded his whiskers, and had grown a pointed beard.

194

He was a distinguished-looking man now, whereas formerly he had only been an impressive-looking one. I do not remember that his stammer was nearly so apparent, and he had far more assurance and dignity. I was still conscious of his great kindness and courtesy, a courtesy distributed with perfect impartiality.

" But the mystery about him is this. The *Life* reveals or seems to reveal a very commonplace man—religious, essentially parochial. His letters are heavy, uninteresting, banal, and reveal little except a very shaky taste in literature. The Essays, which are reproduced, which he wrote for Birmingham literary societies, are of the same quality —serious, ordinary, prosaic, mildly ethical.

" Yet behind all this, this pious, conscientious man of business contrived to develop a style of quite extraordinary fineness, lucid, beauty-haunted, delicate, and profound."

Now does a distiller of vitriol become a distinguished man by fraud and robbery ? I find the clue in the fact that Shorthouse was an epileptic. We know by clinical experience that epileptics may suffer from an extraordinary division of personality. Shorthouse making sulphuric acid in Birmingham and taking high tea was one man. Shorthouse in his study utterly immersed in the seventeenth century was quite another, and one Shorthouse did not know what the other Shorthouse did. The real life and the dream life were separate things, and the initial sentences of his preface indicate a mild surprise at finding a white bird in this nest in the Black Country. In so far as the dream life overflowed into the real life it made a bigger man of him—the complete opposite of Baron Corvo's fate.

But this is the seventeenth century at second hand, and I will merely draw this part of my subject to a close by quoting from an article by John Hayward, which I think puts forcibly and well the decline that accompanied the end of that century.

" The vein of true poetic gold follows a strange uneven course through English poetry, but never more crookedly and unaccountably than in the seventeenth century.

"An age, not 60 years, separates Sir Henry Wotton from Tom Southerne. Sophistication increases as the century draws to its close, though it cannot disguise in a changing world an all too apparent restlessness of thought and sensibility.

"The heaven of Traherne and Herbert, the mystical paradise of Vaughan and Crashaw had passed away ; Herrick's flowers had withered ; in the songs of Dryden and his contemporaries are only echoes of an earlier music ; while the metaphysical brilliance of Donne and Marvell had become dissipated in the absurdities of Cleveland and in Cowley's egregious imitations."

Dryden is not in much favour at the present moment. Professor Housman rated him soundly in his Leslie Stephen Lecture at Cambridge. Speaking of Dryden's attempts to modernize Chaucer, he said : "That there should ever have existed an obtuseness which could mistake this impure verbiage for a correct and splendid diction is a dreadful thought. More dreadful is the experience of seeing it poured profusely, continually, and with evident exultation from the pen of a great and deservedly illustrious author. But most dreadful of all is the reflection that he was himself its principal origin."

He goes on to say : "Meaning is of the intellect, poetry is not. If it were, the eighteenth century would have been able to write it better. As matters actually stand, who are the English poets of that age in whom one can hear and recognize the true poetic accent emerging clearly from the contemporary dialect ? These four : Collins, Christopher Smart, Cowper, and Blake. And what other characteristics had these four in common ? They were mad." He claims that he recognizes the veritable poetic note by its physical effects upon him in the following amusing way : "Experience has taught me, when I am shaving of a morning, to keep watch over my thoughts because, if a line of poetry strays into my memory, my skin bristles so that the razor ceases to act. This particular symptom is accompanied by a shiver down the spine," and so on. "The seat of this sensation," he concludes, "is the pit of the stomach." He here joins hands with Van Helmont across the centuries we have traversed this evening, who located the "sensitive soul" there. It is interesting to find poetry defined in terms of its effect upon the autonomic nervous system, and it again brings us up sharply against authorship, as a conflict between the intellect and the emotions.

Renaissance, Reformation, Rationalism, Romantic Revival, the R's roll on their way, each wave bearing witness to some phase in this eternal conflict. That it is present to-day, smaller wavelets are constantly reminding us. If I select a modern instance, I fear I may not carry you with me as much as I would fain hope I have done so far. For to mention the name of D. H. Lawrence is to see wigs scattered afar upon the green.

Harold Nicolson appears to regard him as the prophet of a new revelation, and thinks that his influence upon the younger generation will in the next few years be overpowering. I rather doubt this. My view is that Lawrence had great literary gifts, which were fatally crippled by his psychoneurosis. And I think that a generation with minds undamaged by the War and the scarcely less disastrous peace which has followed will recognize that fact.

It is generally recognized that D. H. Lawrence was in the grip of mother fixation all his life. So much is clear from his intensely autobiographical novel *Sons and Lovers*, which in my opinion is the only book of his which will prove of permanent value. His mother, disappointed in her husband, turns to her son. In a later book, *Fantasia of the Unconscious*, he had realized the situation and judged it severely. He says : " So she throws herself into a great love for her son, a final and fatal devotion, that which would have been the richness and strength of her husband and is poison to her boy. . . . Parents are the first in the field of the child's further consciousness. They are criminal trespassers in that field. . . . They establish [a] circuit. And break

197

it if you can. Very often not even death can break it."
He clearly recognized, as Middleton Murry said, that
the father failed the mother because he would not
assume purposive responsibility ; the mother failed the
father because she was cold and untender to him ; and
the children were devastated by the diverted and per-
verted love.

Naturally he failed in his adult relationship with
women. Such men always do. He said : " You will
not easily get a man to believe that his carnal love for
the woman he has made his wife is as high a love as
that he has felt for his mother." The word " carnal "
betrays him ; it is all that the mother-fixed can give,
but they ask a great deal more. He met with great
sympathy and help—he recognized that, but could not
avail himself of it. Note this passage : " In her heart the
woman believes that the birth of a child is the appointed
end of sex-fulfilment and the ecstasy only the blossom
on its way to become ripe seed. . . . If she were fulfilled,
according to her own desire, there would be no turning
back, or if there were, it would be only a momentary
turning back of which the man need not be afraid.
But he is afraid : and the fear turns to hate." From his
writings " we fall into the habit of thinking because
Lawrence was so constantly concerned with sex that he
loved it ". Really " it is a fetter which he longs to shake
off. He has the intense hatred felt by the medieval
monk against the humiliation and the cause of it—
woman ". Naturally his wife resents this. " That the
man should regard her as the creature and embodiment
of *his* darkness horrifies her, she repudiates it utterly.
Really he was practically impotent and wanted to be as
a child seeking security and happiness from a protective
woman, but he imagined himself as the hardy, indomitable
male, demanding complete submission. Incapable of
normal sex fulfilment he seeks abnormal fulfilments. But
even in his earlier works the note of homosexuality is
heard, before it becomes explicit in his later novel
Aaron's Rod, where Lilly (who is Lawrence scarcely

198

disguised) wants a homosexual relation with Aaron to complete his incomplete hetero-sexual relation with his wife. This he calls ' extending marriage '. Other people might find a different name for it " (Murry).

Naturally when a man reaches a stage like this he has to try and construct a philosophy to rationalize his abnormal cravings. Hopelessly divided between his sexual appetites and his spiritual love for his mother's memory, while yet knowing how it has destroyed him, he portrays growth as duality, i.e. an increasing cleavage between the senses and the spirit. A tragic if laughable misinterpretation of decay for growth. Frustrated in his relationships with women and men alike, longing to be free without the courage to achieve freedom, his power motive grows to phantastic dimensions ; he must dominate utterly. He talked of " the deep fathomless submission to the heroic soul in a greater man " (meaning himself), and again : " Men must submit to the greater soul in a man for their guidance and women must submit to the positive power-soul for their being." He must go away with a chosen man to make the nucleus of a new society. He must deny reason, find release in mindless sensuality (his own phrase) and find it among pre-mental primitive people. And so he goes forth : first to the Alban Hills, then to Sicily, thence to Sardinia. In each in turn he finds El Dorado—for about a week. For he found that " the mindless human being is malevolent ". He was invited to stay at the Benedictine Monastery at Monte Cassino. His description of his stay is vivid : " They were the old-world peasants still about the monastery, with the hard, small bony heads and deep-lined faces and utterly blank minds, crying their speech as crows cry and living their lives as lizards among the rocks, blindly going on with the little job in hand the present moment, cut off from all past and future, and having no idea and no sustained emotion, only that eternal will-to-live which makes a tortoise wake up once more in spring, and makes a grasshopper

whistle in the moonlight nights even of November."
From the heights of Monte Cassino he looked down again
on to the modern world. " And here above . . . we were
in the Middle Ages. Both worlds were agony to me.
But here on the mountain-top was the worst : the past,
the poignancy of the not-quite dead past."

" I think one has got to go through with the life down
there—get somewhere beyond it. One can't go back "
he said.

And so he passed from disillusionment to disillusionment.
In Sicily he felt that it would be best to be one of the
suave and completely callous demons ; but unfortunately
he could not stand their company. He found that
the Sardinians " have not passed beyond democratic
uniformity, they have not reached it. They are beneath,
not beyond, the civilization which is as necessary to
Lawrence as to any other man who has inherited it ".
And so, like the Wandering Jew, he is driven on and on.
He went to the United States, but as his head was full
of Aztecs and the novels of Fenimore Cooper it is not
surprising that disappointment awaited him again.

To paraphrase Middleton Murry—the question was
this : Did he really accept or did he really reject modern
life—the life into which fitfully and weakly, but yet
finally, the spirit of love has entered ? He would not
decide this ; he wanted to be able to proclaim the pre-
mental as an ideal and to denounce it as an experienced
fact. For he knew that a completely achieved mental
consciousness is the distinguishing mark of the modern
world—that which makes it modern. That ideal country
of his would never be found. Unless he could make himself
a whole he would never find the whole of which he could
be a part, yet his desire for leadership continued and
grew, as did his craving for complete submission of others
to his will. But leadership was impossible for a man so
completely divided between love and hatred. And, as
is usual in such a case, hatred became dominant and
death loomed almost as an escape.

It seems to me, however, that in his last writings he

must have got nearer accepting the truth, for he wrote :
" We dimly realize that mankind is one, almost one flesh.
It is an abstraction, but it is also a physical fact. In some
way or other the cotton-workers of Carolina or the rice-
growers of China are connected with me and, to a faint
yet real degree, part of me. The vibration of life which
they give off reaches me, touches me, and affects me all
unknown to me. For we are all more or less connected,
all more or less in touch : all humanity. That is until
we have killed the sensitive responses in ourselves, which
happens to-day only too often." So he came at last to
" accept the Universe " but he had better have done
so earlier. For his physical frame was by now exhausted
by the hopeless struggle of his divided personality. It
is a story as inevitable as Greek Drama—mother fixation
—the splitting of love into physical and psychical components—impotence—and an attempted compensation for
it in a phantastic power motive which became completely
asocial, and so destroyed itself. His writing is exhibi-
tionism, but also an attempt to explain himself to himself
for, as he said, " one sheds one's sicknesses in books—
repeats and presents again one's emotions to be master
of them." Mingled with his turgid philosophy and
preposterous physiology there are passages of really
lovely comprehension of external nature, and flashes of
self-knowledge. But he puts the final verdict on himself into the mouth of one of his characters : " When it
comes to doing anything—you sort of fade out—you're
nowhere."

One of Osler's profoundest remarks was that we all
drag about with us the chains of the original error in
which we were trained. It is a truth with many applica-
tions—not only to D. H. Lawrence but to every one
of us. We are, for good or evil, the resultant of our
heredity and our environment.

Well, that was a platitude, and I seem to see Osler's
quizzical smile across the room as I utter it. So I will
conclude this attempt to do honour to the memory of
a great man. Medicine is proud of him, but we may fairly

claim that medicine alone could have shaped and developed him to be the man he was. " So true it is," as Stephen Paget used to maintain, " So true it is, that it is not we who make our profession, but our profession which makes us."

DR. JEKYLL DIAGNOSES MR. HYDE [1]

It is a great honour to be invited to deliver the Cavendish Lecture for two reasons. I am proud to follow so many distinguished men in this office, and I am glad to have a share in this commemoration of Henry Cavendish, one of the greatest sons of Cambridge, my own beloved Alma Mater. No one ever pursued science with more devotion and single-mindedness than this shyest, most retiring member of the Devonshire family. It has been said of him that he was " the richest among the learned, and the most learned among the rich men of his time ". Yet his own life was of the simplest and he lived for the advancement of knowledge. His researches in chemistry and electricity were characterized by a rare accuracy and finish. It is fitting that medicine which depends so much on those basal sciences should do honour to his memory, even though we realize one hundred and twenty-seven years after his death that we cannot even aspire to his standard of accuracy in our work. It may seem somewhat of a paradox that to commemorate him I should choose a topic dealing with the least accurate, because the newest, of all the branches of medicine. But, like him, we can claim to be explorers of new ground.

A little more than half a century ago the reading public was gripped by the story of Dr. Jekyll and Mr. Hyde which appeared, as I well remember, as a slim paper-covered booklet. Although Robert Louis Stevenson had been writing for several years he had leapt into fame only two years before with the publication of *Treasure Island*. R. L. S. is not much to the modern taste, I fear, but those

[1] The fifty-fourth Cavendish Lecture, delivered under the auspices of the West London Medico-Chirurgical Society, at the Kensington Town Hall on 3rd June, 1937.

of us whom in youth he invited to gaze through magic casements into the fairyland of his imagination are not likely to forget him. Moreover, the medical profession owe to him the most graceful compliment we have ever received.

It is usually said the idea of Jekyll and Hyde came to him in a dream. That is true, but it is only half the truth. His biographer, Graham Balfour, says : " A subject much in his thoughts at this time was the duality of man's nature and the alternation of good and evil ; and he was for a long while casting about for a story to embody this central idea. Out of this frame of mind had come the sombre imagination of ' Markheim ', but that was not what he required." Do you remember how Markheim the murderer listens in his victim's shop to the many clocks ticking out the minutes to his detection ? Then he hears someone coming quietly up the stairs ; the door is opened and he is confronted by his former self. But Stevenson could not find the story he wanted till one night he had a dream. In the small hours of one morning Mrs. Stevenson was awakened by cries of horror from her husband. Thinking he had a nightmare she roused him. He said angrily : " Why did you wake me ? I was dreaming a fine bogy tale." She had awakened him at the first transformation scene, but he found himself in possession of three of the scenes in the *Strange Case of Dr. Jekyll and Mr. Hyde*. He dreamed these scenes in considerable detail, and so vivid was the impression that he wrote the first draft of the story off at a red heat, just as it had presented itself to him in his sleep.

I need only remind you that Jekyll discovered a drug which transformed him into the degraded Hyde and back again at will. As time goes on the transition downwards becomes easier and in time automatic, while the reverse step grows more difficult and finally impossible. If the moral is obvious the art with which it is conveyed is exquisite.

Stevenson often drew his characters from life. The original of Utterson in this story was his father's lawyer ;

Long John Silver of *Treasure Island* was W. E. Henley, the poet, and Attwater of *The Ebb Tide* was Dew-Smith, one of the founders of the Cambridge Scientific Instrument Company. Sir D'Arcy Power tells me that Dr. Jekyll was a composite portrait, greatly modified of course, of Dr. Radcliffe, then living in Cavendish Square, and Dr. Anstie, of Welbeck Street. Radcliffe was a man of fine presence, but whose whole aspect was apt to be distorted by rage ; Anstie was in the habit of experimenting on himself to a dangerous extent with drugs. This condensation of two individuals is a characteristic of dreams.

The point I want to emphasize is that the dream came into a mind already prepared, as indeed all dreams do. The affairs of the day, wish, fulfilment, unsolved problems, eruption from the unconscious, all such things are the stuff that dreams are made of.

It is significant that Stevenson wrote in a letter to his cousin : " The prim obliterated polite face of life, and the broad bawdy and orgiastic or mænadic foundations form a spectacle to which no habit reconciles me." Indeed, it was a contrast to which he frequently turned. *The Travelling Companion* was a story dealing with his sense of man's double being, but it was rejected by the publisher and the manuscript was burnt by the author. Stevenson's latest biographer, Janet Adam Smith, very aptly points out how the City of Edinburgh itself symbolized for him that sense of double being.

" Socially, Edinburgh was to him a double-faced and deceitful city. There was the polite façade, the squares and crescents of the New Town and the suburbs, filled with people who, in his opinion, married, had children, gave dinner-parties, and went to church on Sundays, not because these things were good or kind or honest in their own right, but because they were socially correct. Behind the prim exterior of the New Town there was the roaring, drunken life of the High Street and Leith Walk and the Lothian Road ; and beneath the frock-coats of the most respectable citizens often lurked malice and brutality and dishonesty. Deacon Brodie, an eighteenth-century embodiment of this duplicity, cabinet-maker by day and housebreaker by night, was the subject of one of Stevenson's earliest stories ; and the fable of Jekyll and Hyde has an obvious application to his view of Edinburgh. The realization of the two-sidedness of the city—and, indeed, of human nature in general—struck Stevenson with all the more force because he had been so carefully kept from seeing anything of it as a child or boy."

Indeed, no one with any imagination can fail to be impressed by the vivid contrasts presented by Edinburgh ; " the sight of Highland Hills round a street corner or, at the end of an alley, ships tacking for the Baltic " ; " the building up of the city on a misty day, house above house, spire above spire, until it is received into a sky of softly glowing clouds " ; the castle on its rock, and the grimy smoky trail of the trains through the heart of the public gardens ; somewhat self-consciously the Modern Athens with a tattered hem or murky slums round the old Canongate. At every turn one is reminded of Winifred Holtby's vivid phrase : " We have lost our tails but have not yet grown wings."

It is not surprising that the creative artist was alive to the division of personality before the medical profession, despite the writings of Morton Prince, appreciated its full significance. Sir James Barrie calls his puckish, freakish *alter ego* McConnachie, George Moore called his Moro, whom he blamed for his lapses from good taste. Sir William Osler christened his familiar spirit Egerton Y. Davis, the initial standing for that fellow of infinite jest—Yorick. Any editor who received an article with that signature had best be on his guard and keep a sharp lookout for subtle, hidden, and sometimes Rabelaisian meanings. Kenneth Walker, another medical writer, boasts the possession of at least four personalities. As long as this recognition of dual or multiple personalities is conscious it does no harm. But sometimes this second personality gains the upper hand. Of this I gave two examples in a previous chapter, Baron Corvo and

J. H. Shorthouse ; in the first the results were harmful, while in the second they appeared to be actually beneficial.

To the inheritors of nineteenth century materialistic medicine it was not a welcome discovery that the psyche is a causal factor in disease. " It is the urgent problems of patients, much more than the questions put by scientific workers which have given effective impetus to the newer developments in medical psychology and psychotherapy." As a result, " to-day we have a psychology founded on experience and not upon articles of faith or the postulates of any philosophical system " (Jung).

One of Jung's valuable contributions to psychology is the conception of a collective unconscious shaped by heredity, from which consciousness develops. We as individuals are branches of the great tree of life, and the nearer we go back to the roots the closer we converge. I can see no other explanation of the persistent recurrence of the same ideas not only in art and literature, but in dreams, neuroses, and insanity, where the old mythological themes frequently reappear in modern dress. Jung has hit upon the method of setting his neurotic patients to draw and paint, with remarkable results. Naturally many of them say they are unable to do so, and on the technical side their efforts are not impressive. But the imaginative content of their pictures is both interesting and illuminating, for the buried conflict in their minds often comes to the surface. Moreover, when one sees the same imagery used by a psychoneurotic in England and by a Chinese artist of the seventeenth century, the existence of a collective unconscious is powerfully supported. It is also of great interest to observe that the reductive process of mental disease resulted in the pictures of artists of such technical skill as the late Charles Sims and Sir William Orpen reverting to just the same style as these patients.

Though the unconscious is not so black as it is painted by Freud, it has its dark side. Jung pertinently inquires : " How can I be substantial if I fail to cast a shadow ? I must have a dark side also if I am to be whole." For many primitive races the psyche is identified with the shadow ; hence to tread on a man's shadow is a deadly insult. You will remember Peter Pan's distress at losing his shadow, and that it was his mother substitute, Wendy, who restored it·to him. Barrie's plays are full of such primitive imagery. Although we owe the very word psyche to the Greeks, later they spoke of the psyche in the more limited sense as *sympaidos*, " he who follows behind ". Markheim's sympaidos who followed behind him up the stairs was his former better self. What Coleridge's sympaidos was like may be judged from those lines in the " Ancient Mariner " :—

> " Like one that on a lonesome road
> Doth walk in fear and dread,
> And, having once turn'd round, walks on
> And turns no more his head,
> Because he knows a frightful fiend
> Doth close behind him tread."

In some the unconscious is Ariel, in others Caliban, but in either case the conscious, Prospero, must be in control. If the conscious and unconscious are at war with themselves a psychoneurosis will result. The recognition of such facts renders our psychoneurotic patients more comprehensible to us, and us more helpful to them. Their complexes are always the cause or the effect of a conflict. Sometimes the conflict may be resolved with unexpected results as in a case recorded by Jung. He says : " I know of a pious man who was a churchwarden and who, from the age of forty onward, showed a growing and finally unbearable intolerance in things of morality and religion. At the same time his disposition grew visibly worse. At last he was nothing more than a darkly lowering ' pillar of the church '. In this way he got along until his 55th year when suddenly one night, sitting up in bed, he said to his wife, ' Now at last I've got it ! As a matter of fact I'm just a plain rascal.' Nor did the self realization remain without results. He spent his remaining years in riotous living and in wasting a goodly part of his fortune." Here it was Mr. Hyde who won.

You will observe that I have quoted a good deal from Jung, nor is it surprising that as one grows older his philosophy should have an increasing appeal. I think that Freud's theories of infantile frustration and sexual repression appeal most to the adolescent, and Adler's theory of the drive towards the goal of life to the ambitions and competitions of middle life. Each has much to teach us but one settles down as life goes on with a sense of relief to the more humanistic, broader conceptions of Jung who appears to see life steadily and to see it whole. It may be urged that he is vaguer, and sometimes not quite comprehensible. Well, are our minds capable of comprehending all the mystery of life ? I am reminded of St. Augustine's vision of the child on the seashore who was trying to empty the ocean into the hole he had dug in the sand. It is Jung's striving to express things which are beyond our ken and which elude our attempts to grasp them that is his fascination for me. He is most likely of all others, in my opinion, to reconcile materialism and metaphysics and to restore our sense of values.

On the practical side, however, we English are showing our national gift for compromise and are selecting from the doctrines of each of these three men the material for a sound system of psychotherapy. As we are living beings the foundation must be biological.

For that medicine will have to become increasingly psychological in its approach I doubt not. It is the needs of our time that has led to the development of this new psychology. And if some academic psychologists scoff at it we can make the simple reply—it works. Although it is only in its infancy, its influence is overflowing beyond the confines of medicine into many other fields of thought, just as did Darwin's exposition of the principle of evolution. A compact body of well-informed medical opinion can be a much needed educative influence in a world which seems to be steadily growing more psychologically sick. For the collective unconscious does not merely manifest itself in the individual ; it is manifesting itself increasingly in herd psychology. The World War released passions which, like Frankenstein's monster or the Bottle Imp, refuse to be imprisoned again. Whether the nations will realize this in time is civilization's present dilemma. I do not believe the position is so hopeless as might appear. Think of the profound disillusionment produced by the events following the French Revolution, the Reign of Terror, and the dictatorship of Napoleon. Edmund Burke said : " The age of chivalry is gone . . . and the glory of Europe is extinguished for ever." Wordsworth in his youth welcomed the tumult of new ideas with the enthusiastic cry :

> " Bliss was it in that dawn to be alive,
> But to be young was very Heaven ! "

But he came to be as disillusioned as Burke and retreated from active affairs to seek relief in a pantheistic conception of nature. Both finished as reactionaries. Just so to-day while soberer minds are anxious, many of the young are indulging in heady draughts of Communism, oblivious of the morning after. Things looked as black for Europe then as they do now, but the skies brightened again, as they may do yet.

Before that can happen, however, nations will have to realize that the Hydes are quite adept at concealing their motives behind Jekyll masks bearing such plausible aspects as patriotism, religion of the state, classless society, and the like. For it is with nations as with individuals. It is embarrassing but true that our friends know quite a lot about our characters which we do not know ourselves. There is an old saying that when A converses with B six persons are involved : each as he thinks he is, each as he appears to the other, and each as he really is. It is pretty clear that the man that Rolfe imagined himself to be became the dominant of these three personalities, while Shorthouse grew to be more like what others imagined him to be. It has been suggested that the absence to-day of the heroes who adorned the Victorian age is due to hero-worship going out of fashion. If it is true that nothing succeeds like success, this is largely due to the fact that some characters tend to expand and flower in the sunshine of approbation. It is equally true that the cold blasts of frustration tend to shrivel others up. Then from the ferment of disappointment a new and abnormal individuality comes to be born. A repressed complex may then assume an autonomous existence, just as a virus apparently incapable of independent life assumes extraordinary vitality and powers of growth within the appropriate host. Repression may for a time be successful and this phantasy personality held in check. Then some shock or strain, or perhaps a physical illness occurs which lowers resistance and out pops the second personality and takes command ; a fugue may follow and the individual is found wandering far from home suffering from complete loss of memory. I will illustrate this from some cases in my own experience.

A man suffering from Bright's disease with some arterial degeneration, strayed from home and was found on Wanstead Flats, some twenty miles away, entirely oblivious of his name and address. I found he had renal disease and under appropriate treatment his memory returned completely and even a year later he remained in fair health. I take him to be a man on the verge of involutionary schizophrenia which was precipitated by toxic influences. When these influences were removed his personality was able to function normally. He reminded me of a patient I saw with oinomania, who ordinarily never had any desire for alcohol. One day when crossing over the street in front of the Mansion House he suddenly had an overwhelming craving for drink. The next thing he remembered was twenty-four hours later when he found himself lying on the railway bank near the signal box outside Weybridge Station. This type is quite distinct from the one where the irresistible craving does not come on till after the first drink. It is generally considered to be due to an unpleasant emotion arising from the unconscious which past experience has shown can be drowned by drink. The memory of the original cause of the emotion has been repressed and the entire response to it has become a conditioned reflex. In the first case the fugue was the result of uræmic toxins acting on a brain with impaired circulation, in the second a repressed emotion was the cause of the intoxication.

A sturdy common-sense Yorkshireman, whom I had seen on and off for several years for mild non-progressive nephritis came into my consulting room one Tuesday and said, " I've lost myself." In response to my inquiry as to his meaning, he told me that on the previous Saturday he came out of his office, saw his car awaiting him but did not get into it, telling his chauffeur that he was going to get his hair cut first. The next thing he remembered was reaching home late at night very cold and exhausted and quite unable to give an account of himself. He stopped in bed the next two days and completely recovered physically but still unable to remember. When I saw him he was clearly frightened by this loss of memory and not pretending. Under light hypnotism he saw himself coming out of the hairdresser's and taking the Tube to Ealing. " Why Ealing ? " I said, knowing that he lived in Palmer's Green. Then it transpired that a woman cousin lived there who knew the business which had been founded by their respective fathers. That morning he had suddenly discovered that his manager had peculated to the extent of £2,000 and left him to face an immediate demand for £1,300 for an account which he believed had already been paid out of the £2,000. But why had the memory of this visit to seek advice and consolation from his cousin faded so completely ? I discovered that his wife disliked hearing of his business worries and equally disliked his cousin's ability to help him over them. The lapse of memory enabled him to get the help without any dispute with his wife. For the time being the division of personality must have been fairly complete, for he apparently discussed the business situation quite rationally with his cousin ;

and had, on the morning of the day when I saw him, acted on the advice she had given, without remembering who had given it till his memory was restored. Here, I think, the toxic element was quite slight.

An able young man in the diplomatic service was liable to attacks of petit mal, which of late had been getting worse, probably associated with disappointed love. His attacks now began to take this form—on reading a novel he would so completely identify himself with one of the characters that he would start up from his chair and act the part of that character ; then he would fall to the ground in a fit of grand mal. Psychological explanation and small doses of luminal greatly improved him and restored his self confidence, while the cure was completed by a happy marriage with another girl. I saw him a year ago quite well and rapidly advancing in the service. He has had no recurrence for the last twelve years.

I have chosen this series to illustrate the grades between toxic and psychogenic factors in the amnesia. For a full discussion of the dissociation of a personality I must refer you to Morton Prince's well-known book with that as its title. There he relates in detail the extraordinary case of a lady whose individuality could change into any one of three different personalities, which he termed respectively the Saint, the Woman, and the Devil, each exhibiting different views, temperaments, and memories. Two of these personalities had no knowledge of each other or of the third, so that in the memory of each there were blanks corresponding to the times when the others were in the flesh. Of a sudden one or the other would wake up to find herself, she knew not where, and ignorant of what she had said or done a moment before. Only one of the three had any knowledge of the life of the others.

Prince remarks that a more correct term would be disintegrated personality, for no one secondary personality preserves the whole psychical life of the individual. The original ego is broken up and shorn of some of its characteristics and memories. The conscious states that still persist synthesize into a personality capable of independent activity, as I suggested under my simile of a virus action. Such disintegration is not identical with degeneration, for it is only a functional dissociation of that complex organization which constitutes a normal self, and which can be reassembled. And so we reach the somewhat platitudinous conclusion that a well integrated personality, one which is not at war with itself is the most capable of withstanding the shocks of physical or psychical trauma.

Of things such as these *Jekyll and Hyde* is an allegory. Just as the sympathetic nervous system works through hormones and the sensori-motor system through simple and conditioned reflexes, so does the mind work through symbols. When you come to think it out you may be surprised to find how symbolical much of our ordinary language is. Fowler in his *Modern English Usage* says that every allegory is a parable and every parable an allegory ; the object of a parable is to persuade or convince ; that of an allegory is often rather to please. The *Oxford English Dictionary* defines an allegory as an extended or continued metaphor. A metaphor is a compressed simile. Now as Fowler says, some metaphors are living, i.e. are offered and accepted with a consciousness of their nature as substitutes for their literal equivalents, while others have been so often used that speaker and hearer have ceased to be aware that the words used are not literal ; but the line of distinction is a shifting one. We constantly mix dead metaphors but we must not mix living ones. Thus if I say to you : " My aim is to construct a theory," I have mixed three dead metaphors without offence. Yet an aim is literally a mark on a target, to construct is to pile up, and the original meaning of theory was " viewing ". If I said " The mark on my target is to pile up a viewing " it would sound nonsense, so metaphorical has our use of those words become. On the other hand, when a journalist wrote : " These are the notes which are most consistently struck in the stream of letters now printed day by day for our edification in the —— " but I forbear to name the paper, and merely quote Fowler's devastating comment, " It is ill playing the piano in the water." Those metaphors still have some life in them and will not blend. But even Fowler, that diligent detective of linguistic errors, omits the further comment that edification is literally a process of building, and that you cannot promote building by playing the piano in a stream. For edification has become a dead metaphor. Even as Homer sometimes nods, so Shakespeare may mix his metaphors, for despite Hamlet we should not be able " to take arms against a sea of troubles " with any real effect. But I have said enough to show how symbolical is our everyday conversation and would warn you that if you watch the habit too closely it may paralyse your powers of speech. It is better to let dead metaphors rest quietly in their tomb.

As in small things, so in greater—in both the mind works in symbols. Much of our misunderstanding of the viewpoints of other ages is due to some shifting in the significance of the symbol. We do not attach quite the same meaning to the words they did in the past, so that the symbol becomes worn like a coin which has been so long in circulation that all its inscription is lost. Yet it is still valid currency. I will conclude by illustrating this from an old symbol and an ancient allegory.

About three years ago I saw a representation of *Cymbeline* at the Festival Theatre, Cambridge, which seemed to me bad and irritating. I was particularly exasperated by the centre of the stage being occupied by the pattern of a labyrinth. Some characters had to thread this maze, others could step over it. What was in the producer's conscious mind I do not know, but I think I comprehended what arose from his unconscious, when I recently read something Mr. Jackson Knight has to say of the ancient ritual maze, such as was found inscribed on a slab in a prehistoric tomb in Anglesea and various other parts of the world. The ritual maze was held to create a field of magic force through which friends could pass while enemies or evil spirits could not. Thus the symbol became an appropriate illustration, even if a rather tiresomely mannered one to a play dealing with the struggle between ancient Britons and the Romans. You will observe that this slab was found in a tomb to exclude enemies from and admit friends to the spirit of the departed. Mr. Knight relates both the labyrinth and the tomb with a world-wide allegory in what is to me a fascinating manner.

The story of the descent of the hero into the under-world recurs again and again in myth and literature. Now in the sixth book of the *Æneid*, Virgil describes Æneas as having been summoned by his dead father to come down to the place of the departed, there to receive counsel as to his future. He arrives at the gate of the Cumæan Sibyl, the doors of which are panelled in relief with the story of the Cretan Minotaur and his victims, and the labyrinth where he devoured them ; a primitive legend of bestiality and human sacrifice. One panel was still empty. We must note in passing that the word labyrinth is derived from labros, the two-headed axe which was the symbol of the rulers of Crete, and was applied to the complicated passages still to be seen in the Royal Palace at Cnossos. To the Greeks this legend symbolized the hostile naval power of Crete which made such depredations on their shores and which they had to make sacrifices of youthful soldiers and sailors to over-come. Virgil was deeply versed in Greek mythology, and it is extraordinarily interesting to find him joining hands with palæolithic man in associating the maze and the tomb. The same story is told in an ancient Sumerian epic and by the natives of the New Hebrides. The collective unconscious again. But to go on with the story itself ; while he is studying these carvings the Sibyl appears. " This," she remarks with some asperity, " is not the time for picture-gazing. You had better get on with your religious duties." Mr. G. M. Young makes this interesting comment : " Taken as a whole and compared with the sculptures on the temple front of Delphi [the carving] is of an earlier, more barbaric, time. . . . ' The sights you are looking at,' the Sibyl means, ' do not belong to our age.' " A new dispensation was at hand ; the day of the

Minotaurs, Hydras, Centaurs, Chimaeras, and the barking Anubis was over and monstrous gods of every form were to be put to flight. For this reason the Roman Church has always put Virgil among the foretellers of the coming of Christ, though it is equally if not more probable that he was referring to Augustus, whom he regarded as the saviour of civilization from the threatened ascendancy of such hideous deities. For Christianity itself was still to have a hard fight in the second century with Mithras and his bull, and indeed had to assimilate some of his tenets.

The empty panel on the gate was left for the future, for the new dispensation to carve with symbols appropriate to higher ideals. So Virgil, that sensitive, hesitant dreamer, imagined, and so we may read in his allegory a message for to-day. Again civilization seems at the parting of the ways ; the monstrous gods of old are hammering on the Gate of the Sibyl ; the darker side of the collective unconscious is assuming a volcanic energy. If it is not to prevail, we must live up the Greek maxim, " know thyself," or Caliban will reconquer the island he inherited from Sycorax, his mother. Dr. Jekyll must diagnose Mr. Hyde by recognizing his origin. Am I too optimistic in hoping that the profession to which Jekyll belonged can by psychological insight play an important part in leading the way to a calmer, humaner, and more rational world ?

THE BACKGROUND TO HARVEY [1]

On 21st June, 1656, William Harvey made his second generous gift to this College, and at his behest the Fellows assembled for the first time to commemorate our benefactors and to heed certain exhortations which by long usage have acquired the significance of a bidding prayer.

Before the next Anniversary came round, Harvey's own blood had ceased to circulate, as Baldwin Hamey expressed it in none too Ciceronian Latin. Thus the second Oration was delivered under the shadow of a great loss ; it may be that in this way the custom arose for it to take the form of a eulogy of Harvey, though this was clearly not intended by the founder.

Although 280 years have passed since the Harveian Oration was instituted, this is, as far as I can determine, the 217th time it has been delivered. As the line of Orators lengthens, the duty increases alike in honour and in responsibility, even though until 1864 the Oration was veiled in what has now become the decent obscurity of the Latin tongue. I am deeply grateful to you, my Lord President, that you should have entrusted me with so honourable, albeit so difficult a task.

The personality of every great man has a certain impact on his own generation, but when Thomas Hobbes said that Harvey was the only man who had seen his theories accepted during his lifetime, he must have been thinking of the younger generation which had grown up since the theory became known. For the men of Harvey's own standing were never convinced. Questions that we know were put to an unsuccessful candidate for the

[1] The Annual Harveian Oration delivered before the Royal College of Physicians on 19th October, 1936.

218

Licentiateship in 1632 prove that his discovery had not yet been accepted by his colleagues. Nevertheless, had his biography been written in the vogue now only too prevalent, of searching for what was called " the real man ", which means a hunt for his failings, Harvey would have emerged from the ordeal very well, and it would still have to be allowed that he profoundly influenced physiology, if not medicine, for the rest of the century.

Mr. Wilfred Trotter said of John Hunter : " It needs all our imaginative sympathy to picture the twilit country in which his labours were carried on—the air is dim and thick, the range of vision short, the appearance of things ambiguous. . . ." This is even truer of Harvey, but as Mr. Trotter pointed out, Hunter's influence was more limited to the indirect and germinal, while every student of physiology is in some sense the beneficiary and direct legatee of Harvey.

I do not aspire to paint yet another portrait of Harvey, for the hastiest perusal of the Orations will prove how well that has been done, but to try and picture something of his background, in the hope that thereby I may do something to make his figure stand out more clearly against it. Not so much the physical background of Cambridge, Padua, St. Bartholomew's, and this College as the background of the thought of his time. An ambitious task, but it has always interested me to inquire why men thought what they did when they did. And this shall be my offering to a great name.

I am the more encouraged to make this attempt because, for reasons I hope to analyse, the seventeenth century has a topical interest for us to-day. Different ages have been interested in different epochs : our fathers were interested in the Renaissance, the Renaissance was interested in the classical age ; to-day we seem to be rounding off a school of thought that was born in the seventeenth century, and so we turn back to inquire, why did men think what they did then ?

We are learning that the dark ages were not so dark

219

as they were painted. The marvellously rapid flowering of the Renaissance tends to blind us to the subtle changes that were occurring before. Sometimes there comes a Spring so early in the year that we fear the return of a frost that will nip the incautious buds. Something of that sort happened in Europe in the thirteenth century. There was a stir in the air. True there had already been a revival of architecture but now a new and delicate art was being revealed by such men as Duccio and Giotto. A new attitude to the world, a frank love of nature, of life in all its manifestations, made its appearance. I like to think it was due to St. Francis of Assisi. His example certainly inspired Giotto to his earliest creative efforts, and the Franciscans were the first scientific investigators of this new age. For when man begins to wonder he desires to investigate. Was not Roger Bacon, the father of English natural science, a Franciscan ?

And then came the frost, and the icy fetters of theological authority imposed a return of winter. Roger Bacon languished in prison for many years and no attempt was made to revive any interest in experiment until the days of his greater namesake. The impulse towards a newer, freer, attitude to life was nipped in the bud and had to throw down deeper roots before again emerging. One great and permanent gift remained—the Universities.

The Renaissance was late in reaching England. Even in France it was unknown till 1494, and the first Renaissance architecture in England is to be found in a Chantry dating from 1500 in Christchurch Minster. In Italy that wonderful efflorescence had found a soil already fertilized as the work of Donatello, Fra Angelico, and Luca della Robbia testified. It has been said somewhat sardonically that at Cambridge " learning like a stranger came from afar " in the person of Erasmus in 1510. Eight years after that Thomas Linacre induced Henry VIII to found this College, and two years later he himself founded lectureships at Oxford and Cambridge, while in 1540, the Regius Professorships were established there. With such a splendid start it may seem strange that the immediate results were disappointing. Yet on inquiry it is not so surprising. For the aim was to revive the old medical learning. It was authoritarian. Medical teaching at the Universities consisted in the reading and expounding of Hippocrates and Galen, and in this College in 1559 John Geynes was cited for impugning the infallibility of Galen. Not until he had humbly recanted was he admitted to our Fellowship in the following year. Something more was needed than the revival of the old ; a new spirit was required to make these dry bones live. It seems paradoxical that the reign of Mary Tudor should have indirectly contributed to this desirable end, but those who fled then to Geneva, Frankfort, and Strasbourg returned on Elizabeth's accession, bringing with them a wider culture than England had previously known. But that new spirit found clearest expression in Francis Bacon's *Novum Organum.* In these days, when every week some book is proclaimed as epoch-making, it sounds jejune to apply this epithet to a work which showed the way to the investigation of the world of phenomena. Projected in his youth, it was prepared by a series of sketches, revised and rewritten at least twelve times, and finally published in 1620.

Men did not realize its portent at once. Even Harvey was mildly scoffing at his distinguished patient's philosophy though he admired the man. Yet as Sir William Hale-White clearly showed in his Oration, he must have been deeply influenced by it. Just so, though more openly, men scoffed at Darwin, Lister, and Freud, only to find themselves, a few years later, utilizing their ideas and their methods. Why does this history repeat itself so inevitably ? Because " there can be no approach to truth without some threat to the thinker's personality " (Trotter). Bacon's dogmatic rationalism of the sciences has never been deliberately followed in its entirety by others. Two, perhaps three, flaws in it may offer a partial explanation. In the first place the defects in his own scientific equipment led to a certain crudity in his conceptions of nature, which gives some justification for Harvey's scoff that Bacon "wrote philosophy like a Lord Chancellor". In the second place he claimed that his way of discovering sciences went far to level man's wits and left little to individual excellence. Never was there a greater fallacy. It leaves out of consideration the scientific use of the imagination. Fabricius had observed the valves in the veins, but regarded them as pockets designed to catch blood that would otherwise have collected in the extremities. Robert Boyle tells us that Harvey saw a tiny but momentous flaw in the argument. For he observed that the veins to the head also had their valves set towards the heart. There was the germ which, cultivated by his scientific imagination, flowered into his immortal discovery. Pasteur said that chance only visits the mind that is prepared. Although Darwin claimed to have worked on true Baconian principles he wrought better than his master knew, for his collection of instances was guided by a hypothesis of which the validity could be tested. No one who has had to disburse the endowments for research can accept the view that the scientific method levels men's wits.

In the third place when Bacon said : " I only sound the clarion, but I enter not into the battle," he deprived himself of the crucial test of his own method. He did as a matter of fact carry out a few experiments, one of which was fatal, for on a wintry day in March, 1626, he caught the chill which ended his life while stuffing a fowl with snow to see if cold would delay putrefaction. It was probably this scant practical experience which led him to slight William Gilbert's work, a more careful study of which would have saved him from some errors. Gilbert was " the first real physicist and the first trustworthy methodical experimenter " and we are proud that he, who influenced Harvey, was a President of our College.

Nevertheless, Bacon " did more than anyone else to help to free the intellect from preconceived notions ". In his own words he pointed the way to " a new and unexplored kingdom of knowledge within the reach and grasp of man, if he will be humble enough and patient enough to occupy it ".

But he was notoriously a better guide in science than in morals and it is impossible to understand seventeenth-century thought without taking into account its pre-occupation with morals. As I urged in an earlier chapter, the Renaissance men felt released from the moral and religious codes which had bound them for centuries ; they believed that they could reap where they had not sown. The subtle awakened intellects appreciated the advantage of brain over brawn and proceeded to exploit the simpler minded. Caius even came to doubt the wisdom of his benefactions and of his support to the new learning. However, the reign of the Machiavellis was not unchallenged for long. Morality would keep breaking through. Over this line of cleavage Shakespeare brooded. A new sensibility was being born and he was conscious of a note of irresolution. He realized that the Mercutio of the south was giving way to the Hamlet of the north. It takes a poet to plumb a poet's mind, and it was John Keats who put his finger on one of Shakespeare's greatest character-istics, his capacity for " being in uncertainties, mysteries, doubts, without any irritable reaching after fact and reason ".

England was awaking from her heady dreams that followed the successful overthrow of the Armada and was beginning to sober down. Though Shakespeare could remain with his mind in suspense, his fellows could not. They wanted facts. Again the cry arose " What is Truth ? " but this time the jesting Pilates stayed for an answer. " The climate of opinion " is a happy phrase we owe to Joseph Glanvill, of Scholar Gipsy fame. How did men comport themselves in the new climate that was surrounding them ? According to their kind ; some simply looked back with bitter regret, others forward with eager anticipation, some imitated Mr. Facing-both-ways.

Richard Burton looked back. He was a scholiast born out of due season, and grew old in an age he condemned. Like the melancholy Jaques in many ways, he had a melancholy of his own, compounded of many simples indeed, for his *Anatomy* is a mosaic of quotations. Mark Pattison described the typical scholastic attitude thus : " If a great writer has said a thing, it is so." It reminds one of case-made law, always so foreign to the medical mind. But the authoritarian note was no longer acceptable in the new atmosphere and Burton felt that by any human standard the entire order of the universe was irrational. It has been said that he was filled with hatred, scorn, and derision for the whole scheme of things in which he found himself. What could one do, he protested with tears in his eyes, but laugh ? Touchstone and Jaques in one.

John Donne, the famous Dean of St. Paul's, on the other hand, illustrates alike in his life and thought the transition from the sixteenth to the seventeenth century. He was " in certain aspects of mind and training the most medieval, in temper the most modern of his contemporaries ". As Mr. John Sparrow wrote with deep insight while still at Winchester, " despite all vicissitudes of fortune, despite even the apparent changes in his character, Donne himself was always essentially the same. . . . There are two ways of arriving at the pitch of emotion necessary for the production of such writings as Donne's. One is the absolute surrender to pleasure and the sacrifice of the ordinary standard of morals ; the other is the complete banishment of pleasure and the consistent living up to an ideal. Donne adopted both of these. . . ." And " there lingers about him something unexorcized, as if Pagan incense were burning in a Christian crypt ".

Brought up a Roman Catholic, he had become Anglican by the time he was 24, but his steps to the altar were somewhat devious and faltering. He was worldly and time-serving, ascetic and devout, with equal sincerity. He stood haughtily apart from his contemporaries except Ben Jonson, for he had the scornful indifference of the innovator regarding himself as destined to inaugurate a new era. He revolted against the conventional and classical imagery of the Renaissance, and was as determined to break it up as Wordsworth was to release poetry from Miltonic diction when it had become outworn through sedulous imitation. Donne experimented with prosody and rhythm like our own Laureate Fellow, Robert Bridges. It is significant that there has been of late a great revival of interest in Donne, just as there has been in El Greco. The writings of one have affinity with the paintings of the other. Both can be ascetic and devotional, just as they can be distorted, startling, and bizarre. This reawakened interest is comprehensible if I am correct in my thesis that certain trends of the seventeenth century are re-asserting themselves to-day. " Every young poet to-day would like to write like Donne ; intensity is the most admired of all qualities. Yet— and there's the rub—so few know what to be intense about—except negative attitudes " (Desmond MacCarthy). Certain it is that modern poets have abandoned the mellifluous line of Tennyson for a condensed allusiveness, an obscurity, a concentration of thought, an imagery drawn from things of everyday life, just as Donne departed from Marlowe's mighty line to the same end. Whether beauty has been served thereby must be left to individual opinion. The modernity of Donne's ideas in some ways is shown by the fact that in 1624, he wrote an essay in favour of voluntary euthanasia. The essence of his intimate thought is to be sought, however, in his *Devotions on Emergent Occasions*, written during a serious illness. Did any writer ever relish an illness so keenly ? It certainly gave opportunity for his self-flagellating temperament, and it is entertaining to observe how gratified he was when the King sent his own physician to consult upon his case.

A greater and more sympathetic figure than either Burton or Donne was Sir Thomas Browne (1603–1682). Like a two-headed Janus he looked both back and forwards. To this peculiarity of his temperament one of the fascinations of his style is due, for it will be observed how frequently a classical phrase or allusion is balanced against an Anglo-Saxon word or homely illustration. Moreover, this dualism of phraseology is accompanied by a dualism of thought, which he clearly acknowledged when he said : " Thus is Man that great and true Amphibium, whose Nature is dispos'd to live, not only like other creatures in diverse Elements, but in divided and distinguished worlds."

To this point of view modern philosophy is tending. The materialistic science of the nineteenth century is dead, neo-vitalism died with the recent lamented passing of its greatest exponent, and while the mechanistic theory of life is being pushed further than ever, its protagonists gladly admit that at most it can only attain one aspect of the truth. Thus Sir Thomas Browne joins hands with the twentieth century, though the way in which he expresses this attitude of his mind may give one the impression of scepticism hand-in-hand with credulity. As he said : " Where truth seems double-faced, there is no man more paradoxical than myself," for he had realized that where a fact or opinion previously widely adopted can be tested by experiment and is not proved correct thereby, you should give it up. But where it is not open to experiment or that method has as yet been insufficiently applied, you are at liberty not to give it up and to doubt the wisdom of those who do. Unlike Bacon, who rejected hypotheses, he attempted to use them. The particular fact was important in Bacon's eyes, the general principle in Browne's.

Sir Thomas Browne was an Honorary Fellow of this College, but it is not correct to say, as is often said, that he became a Fellow of the Royal Society. The name " T. Browne " modestly squeezed into a corner of their Roll is that of his beloved grandson, to whom he wrote such charming letters.

It has been stated on Wilkin's authority that Sir Thomas wrote the Harveian Oration for his son Edward to deliver. The Sloane Manuscripts contain this Oration in Sir Thomas's writing with references to the lecture theatres in different continental universities which

Edward had visited, for on this subject, as his father pointed out, he could tell " more than any other is like to say ". But as a matter of fact Edward was never Harveian Orator. Perhaps with fatherly pride he had expected him to be, and it is unfortunate that he did not live long enough to see his son occupy our Presidential Chair, which would have more than compensated for any earlier disappointment.

It was Sir Thomas Browne who enriched our language with the word " electricity ". That he was himself an experimentalist can be seen from his *Miscellaneous Writings*. Mr. Geoffrey Keynes says that he " may be justly compared with his contemporary Robert Boyle in his restless curiosity and his use of the experimental method, though he fell far short of Boyle in his achievement ". Dr. Joseph Needham, however, attaches great value to his work on the chemical aspects of embryology which has been quite overlooked, although his originality and genius in this field is hardly less remarkable than in so many others. Harvey's approach to embryology, unlike Sir Thomas Browne's, was in the main morphological, and to-day the biochemical aspect of that subject has pride of place.

On such an occasion as this when we are striving to find " an antidote against the opium of time " Browne's " Urne-Buriall " may strike us with a sudden chill— " The iniquity of oblivion blindly scattereth her poppy, and deals with the memory of man without distinction to merit of perpetuity. . . . Diuturnity is a dream and folly of expectation." Yet it is not entirely true, for were it so should we be listening to his solemn music to-day?

Saintsbury, no mean judge, speaks of : " The mixture of shaded sunlight and half illuminated gloom which makes the charm of his style and habit of expression ; its connection with the singular clarity and equity of his temper and judgment is quite unmistakable." How well this corresponds with the description of the man by his intimate friend Whitefoot : " He was never seen to be transported with mirth or dejected with sadness."

He was indeed himself the Great Amphibium, and while he was floating placidly in divided worlds, the great Leviathan pushed on stormily towards a completely materialistic philosophy.

Thomas Hobbes was born in the year of the Armada, and lived through the Civil War, the Commonwealth, and the Restoration to within nine years of the Revolution. Much had he seen and known of changes during those more than ninety years, yet he remained unchanging, obstinately set in his opinions. When the Long Parliament began to be active, he fled to France, where he became tutor to the future Charles II. But in 1657 he returned to England because he feared the attitude of the French clergy, who were no more tolerant towards him than the Puritans.

He was a friend of Ben Jonson, of Lord Herbert of Cherbury, whose philosophy was diametrically opposed to his, of Descartes, and he knew Galileo. Harvey left him a legacy. He was not only a friend of Bacon's but acted for a time as his secretary. Yet he never set much store by experiment, and he founded his mechanical theory on Galileo rather than on Bacon. It is a little disconcerting to find that men of such varied culture left him so unaltered. It is also suggestive of some attractive traits in the man that they put up with his truculence. His theory was neither attractive nor flattering, starting as it did from a belief that the whole nature of man is a consistent scheme of selfishness. It was not until he was 40 that he formulated his philosophy on a geometrical basis. I like Aubrey's account of this. In a friend's library " a copy of Euclid lay open at the forty-seventh proposition of the first book. So he reads the proposition. ' By God,' says he, ' That's impossible.' So he reads the demonstration which referred him back to another (and so on) that at last he was demonstratively convinced of that truth. This made him in love with geometry ". He wanted to reduce the doctrine of justice and policy in general to the " rules and infallibility of reason after the fashion of mathematics ". For him motion was the one reality, all

others but " the fancies, the offspring of our brains ".
From geometry he passed through physiology to moral
philosophy, believing that " the motions of the mind have
physical causes ". There is a suggestion of conditioned
reflexes and behaviourism in the statement that " the
internal motions set up by the action of objects upon the
sense become reactions on the external world and these
reactions minister to the preservation of the individual ".
He maintained that the appetites and passions of men are
such that unless thay be restrained by some power they
will always be making war upon one another. Government is a social compact for the sake of peace, and men
must give up their rights to one man or one assembly
of men. And thus we arrive at the absolute monarch, who
has rights but no duties, as the apex of this pyramid.
Curiously modern some of these items, even if the sequence
is a little obscure : matter as a form of motion, and
conditioned reflexes leading up to the conception of a
totalitarian state. And this quotation is painfully topical :
" Covenants of mutual trust where there is a fear of not
performance of either part are invalid." These are the
main arguments in his chief and most famous book
The Leviathan. But though an amateur he could not
refrain from controversy with genuine mathematicians
and scientists such as John Wallis, the first of Glisson's
pupils to proclaim Harvey's discovery in public and with
the great Robert Boyle. In these disputes he was labelled
" the greatest of circle-squarers ".

There is a logical sequence in his attempt to show that
the whole fabric of human life and society is built out of
simple elements. It is in his premises that error lies, for
" the individual is neither real nor intelligible apart from
his social origin and traditions [which] influence his
thoughts and motives " (Sorley).

Still, as I have reminded you, certain schools of thought
to-day favour this pushing of the mechanistic theory as
far as it will go, while recognizing, as Hobbes did not,
that it must leave a whole system of values untouched.
And for good or evil the Totalitarian State is with us

to-day. So one cannot help feeling a certain regard for the obstinate old man who stuck to his logic with more than French tenacity and who was only just spared from seeing the divine right of kings finally perish in this country with the landing of William of Orange.

For throughout the century the doctrine of the divine right of kings had been challenged by a people who were finding their staple intellectual and spiritual food in the Authorized Version of the Bible. As Fisher says : " Here was a people's university. Plunging into this vast miscellany, where all that is most solemn and sublime from the distant East is mingled with the records of a savage antiquity, the peoples of England wandered at their own sweet will, unshepherded and unfettered, and finding always by the way lessons for the conduct of life, some of infinite depth and beauty, but others prompting to gloom, pride, and self-sufficiency."

What the nation needed on waking from the heady dreams of the Renaissance was what Europe needs to-day —a time of political peace and social calm. But it was not to be. Though knowledge continued to grow, the thoughts and emotions of the people were diverted by class hatred, religious controversy, and political storms. The climate of opinion was overcast with thunder clouds, and Milton's " two-handed engine at the door " stood ready to smite. It has been well said that it was King James's Bible that cost his son his head.

I believe that if the Cambridge Platonists could have had their way much strife would have been avoided. In the political and theological turmoil of the times their's was a steadying and pacifying influence but unhappily not sufficiently widespread. Yet Harvey thought little of them. In this matter he was more Royalist than the King.

Their home, both spiritual and material, was Emmanuel College. In 1584 Sir Walter Mildmay obtained a charter of incorporation, purchased the home of the Black Friars which had fallen into ruin after the dissolution of the monasteries and rebuilt it as Emmanuel. Mildmay was a

puritan and from the first the college had a decidedly
puritanical character. He told Queen Elizabeth that
" he had set an acorn, which when it becomes an oak,
God alone knows what will be the fruit thereof ". That
acorn grew fast, and Fuller wrote in 1634 : " Sure I am
at this day it hath overshadowed all the University, more
than a moiety of the present masters of Colleges being
bred therein." Soon after Fuller wrote this, the influence
of Emmanuel was to spread across the Atlantic, for
John Harvard migrated thence to Massachusetts and there
with his father's money saved a college from disaster to
make it the pioneer university in the United States.
Mullinger, the erudite, if eccentric, Librarian of St. John's
College in my undergraduate days regarded Sherman of
Trinity as the founder of the movement, and Henry More,
who was certainly a leader, hailed from Christ's. But all
the others, of whom I need only mention Whichcote,
John Smith, Cudworth, and Culverwel, were all trained
at Emmanuel. Their avowed intention was to bring the
Church back to " her old loving nurse the Platonick
philosophy ". Their Platonism was in Wordsworth's
phrase " reason in her most exalted mood ", and has
been expressed more fully as " the mood of one who has a
curious eye for the endless variety of this visible and
temporal world, and a fine sense of its beauties, yet is
haunted by the presence of an invisible and eternal
world behind or . . . within the temporal and visible "
(J. A. Stewart). But they were not mere mystics ; they
regarded abstention from dogmatism as one of the most
effective means of promoting unity and concord.
Whichcote held that the inductive method was as
calculated to prove effectual in allaying theological
contention as it had been in the hands of Galileo and
Harvey in their respective fields. He maintained that
authority proceeds from right reason, not reason from
authority. And further he said : " It ill becomes us to
make our intellectual faculties, ' Gibeonites ', hewers of
wood and drawers of water for the will and the emotions."
No wonder that most of them detested Hobbes's

materialistic philosophy and were alarmed at his influence. Though he was intellectually more than a match for them they had a vision which he lacked.

Though Puritan in origin it would be a mistake to regard them as simply Puritans ; theirs was a middle course. They had that wider culture which is sometimes successfully grafted on a Puritan stock. Dean Inge in his book on the Platonic tradition says : " Besides the combative Catholic and Protestant elements in the churches, there has always been (this) third element with very honourable traditions, which came to life again at the Renaissance but really reaches " much further back. " The flame which [the Cambridge Platonists] kindled among us was lighted in Italy, when Grocyn and Linacre visited the famous Platonic Academy at Florence." But they received " the treatment, as we know both from history and fiction which those must expect who interpose their persons between two violent combatants. . . . In time of war the prophet and seer are not wanted. Effective partisan cries have to be devised which will appeal to and be understood by the masses. All fine issues are coarsened ".

One must regretfully feel that just as the story of the Reformation would have been very different if Erasmus instead of Luther had been its leader, so would the history of Charles I's reign if Roundhead and Cavalier could have listened to the sweet reasonableness of these Platonists. But the scholar is no match for the demagogue at such times.

Yet their labour was not in vain in the intellectual world. Only six months after Henry More entered Milton left Christ's. We know that he described his academic studies as " an asinine feast of sow thistles and brambles " yet a few years later " Cambridge men were deep in Descartes and some of them in Bacon ". A new intellectual life sprang into being and the leaven spread as the Platonists were appointed to responsible positions throughout the University.

I cannot enter the courts of Emmanuel without feeling

that something of the cool restraining influence of those Platonists haunts them still. They should be living at this hour. Peace be to their ashes.

We are apt to forget that all the Athenians were not reasonable enlightened people, clearly though their refusal to learn from experience proclaims the fact. In the same way we sometimes forget that the enlightenment of the Renaissance never penetrated the popular mind, which remained largely medieval in outlook. Just so to-day we can see what the ordinary man feels and thinks from the letters he is impelled to write to the popular press rather than from the writings of Whitehead and Inge. The great Witch controversy of the seventeenth century throws light on the popular mentality, in which, alas, greater minds shared. To us it seems almost incredible that such men as Sir Thomas Browne, Henry More, and Joseph Glanvill should have believed in witches. But we must remember they felt that to doubt the existence of evil spirits implied an equal doubt in the existence of beneficent spiritual forces. In appealing to demonology, they were " tapping a reservoir of traditional super-natural belief which lay deeper in the national consciousness than Christianity itself, and deeper certainly than the new ice-crust of rationalism which now covered it " (Willey). H. V. Routh explains this obsession in terms of modern psychology by saying : " As men struggled towards a higher level of civilization, they instinctively accused these pariahs (witches, etc.) of all that . . . progress had branded as accursed, but could not eradicate from the imagination. . . . For many, and in some cases subconscious motives men wished to believe in witch-craft—and the intellect generally follows the emotions." It was the peaceful penetration of the scientific outlook which ultimately destroyed the belief in witchcraft.

In this matter Harvey was on the side of the angels. We know that he presided over the committee who examined the survivors of the unfortunate Lancashire witches in 1634, and pronounced them free from any of the signs then supposed to indicate a witch. Then there is the amusing story of his being sent by the King to inquire about a witch on Newmarket Heath. Harvey pretended to be a wizard and got her to show him her familiar—a pet toad. In her absence he dissected it and found it to be an ordinary toad. He pacified the old woman, exasperated by the loss of her pet, by explaining he was the King's physician and had adopted this method of clearing her reputation. One can vividly picture the scene ; indeed, if Harvey were the " cholerick little man " as pictured by Aubrey, it is all the more to his credit that he handled the infuriated beldame so gently. Nor does his courtesy in controversy, so rare in those days, support Aubrey's epithet. We may attribute some share in this tolerant attitude of his to the united family that formed the background of his early life. Indeed, throughout they obeyed the request in their father's will to live in unity and mutual help, and one hears an echo of this in Harvey's injunction to our College.

The background furnished by Caius College, St. Bartholomew's Hospital, and our own College has been fully described by others and needs no comment from me save this : we like to think of them in terms of our personal knowledge, but they have all changed, almost beyond recognition, and changed immensely for the better. But until the War Padua still looked much as it must have done when Harvey paced its colonnaded streets and secluded Botanic Garden. He must have gazed on Giotto's simple dignified frescoes in the Chapel of the Arena, and marvelled as we do still at the mingled beauty and learning so enthusiastically expressed by the youthful Mantegna on the pictured walls of the Eremitani. The vast Salone still shelters Donatello's wooden horse and his sculptured high altar reposes under the five domes of San Antonio. In the buildings of the University, nicknamed " Il Bo " stands the anatomical theatre where Harvey watched the dissections of Fabricius ; that theatre which served as the model for the old anatomical theatre at Cambridge that survived into my own student days. Just as the spirit of his maturer age is preserved in

234

this College, so in Padua we can best realize the material surroundings of Harvey's youth. Here, too, we may well imagine he gained that knowledge of art which fitted him to be entrusted with the responsibility of buying pictures in Venice for such a connoisseur as Charles I.

Soon after that historic cannon-ball on Edgehill had roused Harvey from his book he retired to Oxford and the pursuit of embryology. He had previously gathered much practical lore from the keepers of the royal forests, and a countryman said of him : " If he had been as stiff as some of our starched and formal doctors he had known no more than they." It must have been a relief to leave the turmoil behind and to watch the development of the chick in Bathurst's rooms in Trinity. This aspect of his work has quite naturally received less attention in these Orations, except for Dr. Herbert Spencer's scholarly exposition fifteen years ago. Since then embryology has advanced in a new direction which makes it fitting to return to the subject for a few moments.

The widest differences of opinion have been expressed concerning his *De Generatione Animalium*. Sir George Ent felt like " another Jason, enriched with the Golden Fleece " when he was allowed to carry it off for publication. Some others have regarded it as a splendid failure. The recent critical analyses of its contents by Needham and by Meyer will help to restore the balance between those two extremes. One cannot help feeling that loyalty to a great name has inspired the praise lavished by some and that the work contains much speculation as well as observation.

I said at the outset that the personality of every great man has a certain impact on his own generation. The converse is inescapably true. We may rightly marvel more at the release from contemporary thought which Harvey displayed in his work on the circulation than at his bondage to it as shown in his embryology. The results of the different mental attitudes that characterize the two books may be summed up in Bacon's aphorism : " If a man will begin with certainties he shall end in

doubts, but if he will be content to begin with doubts
he shall end in certainties." When at the end Harvey said
he despaired of understanding development, we may
fairly ask whether he did not begin with what he regarded
as some certainties.

Yet much of value remains. Harvey stoutly upheld
the doctrine of epigenesis against the prevalent theory
of preformation. It is astonishing what a hold that Chinese
box idea of the ovum continued to have even into the
early nineteenth century. Harvey's conception of the
gradual differentiation of the simple and homogeneous
into the complex and heterogeneous showed philosophical
insight and anticipated the ideas of the present century.
Nor was this all. He anticipated Glisson by a quarter of a
century in the generalization that all living tissues are
characterized by a response to stimulation, and he
contested the view of his own master, Fabricius, that the
maternal and fœtal circulation directly communicate.
And to him we owe the epigrammatic generalization
" ex ovo omnia ".

Considering how little Cambridge did for Harvey in
his lifetime, I feel in private duty-bound to emphasize
something of what my University has done in the last
sixty years to develop some of his views. Harvey's idea of
the intrinsic rhythm of heart muscle was carried to
triumphant demonstration by Gaskell and has formed the
basis of the new cardiology. Frank Balfour's evolutionary
conceptions of embryology may be out of fashion now, but
what a stimulus they gave to the whole of animal
morphology. And they were based on epigenesis.
Balfour had been dead seven years when I went to
Cambridge but his old department was still lit with the
radiance of his enthusiasm. The studies of Walter Heape
and of our own Baly Medallist, F. H. A. Marshall, have
carried on the torch. And the latest phase, the new
chemical aspect of embryology, is associated with the
name of Joseph Needham, our Oliver-Sharpey Lecturer
of this year.

I have tried throughout to indicate the ways in which

the turmoil of thought in Harvey's time is reproducing itself to-day. In both instances there had been a phase of great and rapid expansion both in thought and in wealth, followed by disillusionment on the intellectual side and greater stringency on the financial. On each occasion old standards were destroyed before adequate new ones could be provided in their place. A new phase of thought is accompanied by a new form of art. If the Baroque did not spring from the Counter-Reformation it was at least greatly fostered by it. The exponents of the new Baroque, Picasso and Epstein, appear to express the feelings of the post-War generation more satisfactorily than they do mine. In their influence on younger poets, Donne is paralleled by T. S. Eliot. It is not without significance that some modern writers are beginning to justify Machiavelli and his ideal of the domination of a ruthless leader, while Elizabethan and Jacobean thinkers felt the effect of his doctrines to be corrosive and withering. It has been well said that " the sinking of the clear exaltation of Elizabethan dramatic poetry into the sophisticated, satirical, conflicting mood . . . of the Jacobean drama had many concurrent causes. The apprehension, regret, and disillusionment inevitable to the conscious passing of a long period of high civilization were not in this case unfounded and those who had known the great age, even those who had only grown to manhood during its latest years were touched by them (like the generation that succeeded the Great War) without being able to define their loss in what had passed. Moreover . . . a stage of development in which some transition from wonder and discovery to assessment and criticism was inevitable ". The modern parallel unfortunately needs no emphasizing. There is, however, one outstanding difference. Then the way of investigation by experiment was new and seemed full of hope ; now there are murmurs to be heard against science itself. Bacon's utterances have not quite the same thrill. The discovery of facts has not in the long run proved so exhilarating after all (Basil Willey). Science on the one hand offers material comfort, on the other intellectual abstractions. This leads to a mechanized world without moral direction. Too many men use dangerous machines like toys as would a child. In the reaction against this we are actually hearing sighs of regret for the passing of the scholiasts, with their strange doctrine that a belief can be metaphysically true though empirically false. Men grasp at the indeterminacy of the atom to revive the idea of miracles. As in other ages of spiritual doubt and political uncertainty, the cult of astrology, not to mention other strange cults, is becoming fashionable.

Man's brain has not been able to adapt itself quickly enough to the material changes of the last hundred years. Sir Alfred Ewing was saddened in his last years by the use men were making of the inventions he himself had helped to promote. Lowes Dickinson asked if there were a way of escape from the alternatives—shall we allow science to destroy us or shall we destroy it to save ourselves ? Such statements, however, relate to the physical sciences—biology must restore the balance. If we would understand ourselves—a much needed investigation—we must realize that we are subject to the laws of biology. A study of history from the biological angle would contribute towards that understanding.

And of all branches of biology, medicine can take the largest share in the reconciliation of science with ethics. In these latter days medicine is becoming increasingly psychological in its approach to suffering, while developing its scientific armament as much as possible. The field of medicine is ever widening ; we can neither remain isolated in our laboratories nor merely stay by the bedside. We are taking a broader view of Harvey's injunction to seek out the secrets of nature and are becoming one of the leading social services. In that development I am proud to think that this ancient College is now playing an increasingly important part.

Towards the end of his life Harvey wrote to a young medical man that as an explorer his own days were, alas, numbered. " But," said he, " it will always be a pleasant sight to see distinguished men like yourself engaged in this honourable arena." There spoke the true spirit of adventure, glad to hand on the torch to the younger generation. In like spirit it is good for us, on this the morrow of St. Luke's Day, to pause amid the rush of life for an hour to join hands with those who have gone before and with those who will come after us. Thus is the real continuity of this College assured.

And so I exhort you in Harvey's own words " for the honour of the profession to continue in mutual love and affection ".

III

SOME GODS AND THEIR MAKERS

SOME GODS AND THEIR MAKERS

When Samuel Butler inverted Pope's aphorism and declared : " An honest God is the noblest work of man," he uttered, not a paradox, but a profound truth. To a large extent every nation has the God it deserves. The kind of God a man desires tells us much of what he is— but tells us even more of what he will become. By their Gods ye shall know them.

I well remember the stir that accompanied the publication of Frazer's *Golden Bough* during my undergraduate days at Cambridge. Here was the first real attempt to make mythology a science. The lovely lake of Nemi assumed a new and even sinister significance. In my schooldays Macaulay's swinging lines—

> " The Priest who slew the Slayer
> And shall himself be slain "

might stir the imagination, but it was left to Frazer to make us realize the inner meaning of that incessant watchfulness, that recurring tragedy in a setting of beauty and apparent peace, as a parable of man's struggles with the forces of life and death, with something awe-inspiring and greater than himself.

That realization has turned some of us back to mythology with a new interest and an intention to discover from it, if we could, the ways in which man sought to interpret, to harmonize and to come to terms with forces and mysteries beyond his ken. And that study has made us realize the remarkable resemblance between mythology and the mentality of savages. We no longer accept the seafaring man's verdict of their manners and customs—" manners none ; customs nasty." We are

243

not so anxious to teach them our manners and we study their customs with interest.

From such studies Frazer has enriched our knowledge of primitive man's mental processes, thereby throwing light upon our own. We can learn something of the process of god-making from his Lectures on the early history of the Kingship, which may be paraphrased thus. At an early stage of society men ignorant of the processes of nature and of our very limited control over them, arrogated to themselves functions which we should deem superhuman. Struck by the marvellous order and uniformity with which nature conducts her operations, the savage was able to foresee them and therefore mistook them for an effect of his own will or, in the case of a dreaded occurrence, of the will of his enemies. In time the fallacy of this belief became apparent, and the unattainable good, the unsuitable ill were next ascribed to the action of invisible powers. Thus magic tends to be displaced by religion, and the sorcerer by the priest. At this stage of thought the ultimate causes of things are conceived as persons, which have not begun to coalesce into a single unknown. Accordingly as long as men look upon their gods as akin to themselves and not raised to an unapproachable height, they believe it to be possible for those of their number who surpass their fellows to attain to divine rank after death or even in life. Like their predecessor the magician, they are expected to guard their people, to heal them in sickness, and to bless them with food and offspring. Men credited with powers so lofty naturally hold the highest places in the land. They are kings as well as gods. Thus the divinity of kings has its roots deep down in human history, and long ages pass before these are sapped by a profounder view of nature and of man. In my Maudsley lecture I dealt with the further evolution of the doctrine of the divine right of kings from the king as a sacrificial object. At Nemi we meet with a mitigation of that custom which allowed the Priest-King to live and reign so long as he could defend himself against all comers in single combat, thus proving that the dreaded decay of his divine powers had not yet set in.

But there is another very important outcome of this doctrine which, like the priest who slew the slayer, tends to kill the doctrine itself. Something higher than the king emerges—law and justice. G. M. Trevelyan has shown very strikingly in his *History of England* how the gradual growth of the Common Law out of fusion of the king's will and local customs developed into something stronger than the king himself. By the time of Charles I this had become powerful enough to challenge the king and even to slay him. Yet even after that a last relic of the superstition of the divine power of English kings lingered in the belief that they could heal scrofula by their touch. Hence the name, King's Evil, for this disease. William III, who certainly could claim no divine right, contemptuously turned away the applicants for his healing touch with a consolatory dole. Only once he laid his hand on a sufferer with the words : " God give you better health and more sense." But Queen Anne resumed the custom, and it is extraordinary to recall the fact that Dr. Johnson, whose rationalism led him to confute Bishop Berkeley by kicking a stone, was himself, as a child, touched for King's Evil by Queen Anne. So hard do superstitions die. Indeed, they lingered on the Continent till 1918, when it was shown that the logic of the stricken field reinforced the sacrificial aspect of kings rather than their divine right. Shakespeare, who saw deeper into the heart of things than any other mortal man, had realized all this long before :—

> " Upon the King ! let us our lives, our souls,
> Our debts, our careful wives,
> Our children and our sins lay on the King.
> He must bear all. Oh hard condition.
> Twin-born with greatness.
>
> .   .   .   .   .
>
> What kind of God art thou, that suffer'st more
> Of mortal grief than do thy worshippers ? "

Wagner represents Wotan as inscribing laws and treaties on the half of his spear by which he himself is bound. But as Bernard Shaw points out—however carefully these laws are framed to represent the highest thoughts of the framers at the moment of their promulgation, before a day has elapsed that thought has grown and widened by the ceaseless evolution of life ; and lo ! yesterday's law has already fallen out with to-day's thought. Yet if the high givers of that law themselves set the example of breaking it before it is a week old, they destroy all its authority with their subjects and so break the weapon they have formed to rule them for their own good. They must, therefore, maintain at all costs the sanctity of the law, even when it has ceased to represent their thought ; so that at last they get entangled in a network of ordinances which they no longer believe in, and yet have made so sacred by custom and so terrible by punishment that they cannot themselves escape from them. Wotan finally began secretly to long for the advent of some power higher than himself, which would destroy this artificial empire of law. As he crosses the rainbow bridge, into the fancied security of Valhalla, where in reality he will only pass into the twilight of the Gods, he dreams of that power as a rescuing hero. He little realizes that one of the first acts of that hero will be to destroy him. For Wotan has gradually and inevitably become separated in sympathy even from his own offspring. " Such a separation is part of the bewilderment that is ever the first outcome of the eternal work of thrusting the life energy of the world to higher and higher organization." " When the Gods arrive the half-gods go." In other words, the progress of thought is always from the concrete to the more abstract. Seen near at hand the concrete image is recognized as only a symbol of something beyond. When this point is neared, men inevitably divide into two parties, one maintaining that the symbol is the real presence, while the other would go always a little farther on the voyage of discovery.

I pointed out in an earlier chapter that there is another

important aspect of this doctrine of the divine right of kings, based on the idea that the king being unlike the common ruck, is possessed of a soul that can achieve immortality ; for it is generally agreed that the great influence of the mystery religions was due to their promise to the common people, also of the attainment of a soul and therefore of immortality.

Everyone who has visited the Baths of Diocletian in Rome is familiar with the beautiful three-sided sculpture in relief, which is usually called the Throne of Aphrodite, though, as the attendant maidens are lifting the goddess from the earth and not from the water, it is clearly Persephone who is portrayed. This delicate relief, which dates from the first quarter of the sixth century B.C., marks the authentic spring-time of Greek art. It bears the same relation to Pheidias that Chaucer does to Shakespeare. All we know of its history is that it was excavated from the site of the garden of Sallust during the Renaissance. Now in 1911, when the effects of an old collector at Lewes were being dispersed, a singular three-sided relief was discovered in his garden. Its origin is quite unknown, its destination was almost certain— America. Most experts are agreed that these two works, separated from one another through so many centuries, were from the same chisel and originally formed one piece. Each is necessary to the interpretation of the other, and taken together they illustrate the Eleusinian Mysteries. Recent excavations at Eleusis go to show that there was a tender and beautiful meaning in the process of initiation there, leading up to the recognition of Θεος, Θεα (Theos, Thea), the divine principle in man and woman. That on their return to Athens the initiates were met at the bridge by their friends with gibe and jest is merely analogous to the unedifying social customs that surround the marriage ceremony to-day. In these mysteries the beautiful myth of Demeter and Persephone was utilized to enforce the significance of renewal of life on the earth, through the symbol of seedtime and harvest, and extended to give hopes of personal immortality in almost the same terms as those subsequently used by St. Paul. Since the cult of Dionysus sprang from the threshing floor, it is not surprising that he played an important part in the rites at Eleusis. His history is a good illustration of the process of god-making. He was a god of the indigenous inhabitants of Greece, while the Gods of Olympus were those of the invading northerners, the representatives of the Iron Age which overwhelmed the Age of Bronze. We can imagine a parallel condition if the Normans had brought their own gods into England, while the Saxons went on worshipping a local tutelary deity. Gradually Dionysus was elevated to Olympus, and all the steps in his apotheosis are shown in the reliefs which support the stage of his theatre at Athens. This apotheosis really symbolizes the steps in the complete fusions of conqueror and conquered.

The prototype of the resurrection gods, who die that they may live again, was Osiris. His sufferings, death and resurrection, were enacted every year at Abydos. In the temple of Isis at Philæ there is a chamber dedicated to him, where he is represented as dead ; out of his body spring ears of corn, while a priest waters the growing stalk from a pitcher. The inscription reads : " This is the form of him whom we may not name, Osiris of the mysteries, who, springs from the returning waters." For just as in other countries the fertilizing rainy season is eagerly expected so, in Egypt it is the flooding of the Nile, the returning waters, which brings about the return of life. At Denderah Osiris is represented first as a mummy lying flat in his bier. Gradually he raises himself, till at last he rises between the outspread wings of Isis, while before him a male figure holds the " Crux Ansata ", the cross with a handle, the Egyptian figure of life. But the God who died and rose again is a world-wide symbol. Such is Balder the Beautiful, the prototype of innumerable St. Sebastians. Ezekiel beheld what he deemed " the abomination " of the " women weeping for Tammuz ". Each year he died and passed below the earth to " the land from which there is no returning ".

The goddess Istar went after him, and while she was below life ceased on the earth, no flower blossomed and no offspring of animal or man was born. In Grecian lands Tammuz became Adonis, " the type of transient loveliness and swift decay." To-day in Palermo we see the Gethsemane gardens set up on Good Friday, which exactly reproduce the gardens of Adonis of pre-Christian days. It was not the beauty of the changing seasons, however, but their influence on the food supply which impressed primitive man. To us a bad harvest may be an inconvenience, but where the ordinary supply falls short food can be obtained from other lands. Not so primitive man ; a bad harvest was a calamity which brought actual starvation in its train. Then the decay of the year spelt death. Small wonder that the anxious anticipation of the Spring, with all its hopes of renewal of the fruits of the earth, was a time of excitement. Small wonder that the harvest festival assumed a religious significance, which it still retains. The tense excitement found its relief in dancing round the threshing floor. A leader of the dance was chosen each year from among the young men, and as time went on and there was a succession of beautiful youths to look back on, at length reaching far back beyond the memory of the oldest inhabitant, it seemed to them that these youths were the earthly representatives of someone in the misty past, a youthful god filled with the wine of life, by whose aid these good things came. And thus Dionysus was born, thus his cult arose. The God sprang from the cult, not the cult from the God. In front of his theatre in Athens still stands the threshing floor, too sacred in the eyes of the Greeks to be destroyed when the cult assumed a more dramatic guise : the threshing floor where these dances took place amid the sound of the flails and the glad rejoicing that plenty had conquered want.

The cult assumed a more dramatic form, out of which the Greek Drama as we know it arose. The orchestra literally means the dancing place, and on the hillside above, the people sat to look on and to enter into the spirit of the scene—from the Θεατρον, the theatre, the seeing place. The leaders were first distinguished merely by the high buskin which raised them above the level of the rest of the chorus, and it was not till later that these leaders were placed more conveniently on a raised platform, the stage. The chorus, which seems to us a rather unmeaning convention, was therefore, in fact, the very origin and kernel of the drama. Æschylus was the first man to introduce two principals in the drama ; Sophocles made use of three. These apparently simple steps were striking innovations in their time, but Æschylus and Sophocles faithfully interpreted the ways of God to man, according to the orthodox belief of the day. Euripides was the questioner of the accepted order, the sympathizer with the under-dog. He saw Athens in peril of change. And then came Aristophanes, the disillusioned mocker, disillusioned by the Peloponesian war. Small wonder, as a writer in *The Times* pointed out, that Æschylus and Sophocles appealed to the Victorians, while the next generation were led by Professor Gilbert Murray to appreciate the extraordinary modernity of Euripides. But now Aristophanes has more appeal. He " was a post-war writer. He wrote for a public suffering from ills which are familiar to us all—an excess of government in all its forms, a contraction of personal liberty, monstrous taxation, a systematic oppression of the middle classes, the supremacy of the *arriviste*, a profound distrust of the democratic experiment." Galsworthy in one respect, Bernard Shaw in another, fill the place of Euripides, while our Aristophanes is Noel Coward. Here, indeed, history is repeating itself, and for similar reasons. Standing in the beautiful theatre of Dionysus, we who have lived through the last quarter of a century can join hands in spirit with the Greeks of the fifth century before Christ. We, too, have watched accepted standards questioned, crumble, and dissolve, and the theatre resounds with the mocking laughter of Aristophanes. Yet while the theatre mocked, Socrates, Plato, and Aristotle were laying new foundations ; a hopeful omen for to-day.

Although Dionysus presided over the theatre and was represented as incarnate there, the orthodox Greeks themselves sometimes complained that the plays performed had " nothing to do with Dionysus ". You, too, may be feeling that all this has very little to do with Dionysus, but it serves to show how the worship of fertility itself raised up a god as its emblem and then overwhelmed the god by the very artistic triumphs his cult originated. As life became fuller, men could not live by bread alone.

In Northern climes the May Queen and Jack-in-the-Green are, of course, survivals of similar cults. But it may not be so well known that on Shrove Tuesday there was, at any rate till recently at Dorking, a football match played in the main street, the two teams being residents east and west of the parish church. In former days the match actually started in the churchyard. There used to be a similar contest at Derby, and still is one at Ludlow. This is the English equivalent of the carnival, and represents the ἀγών or contest. " The simplest form of spring festival takes little notice of death and winter, but in other and severe climates the emotion is fiercer and more complex." The struggle between starvation and the will to live is dramatized as a contest. Thus the Esquimaux symbolize it by a tug-of-war between ptarmigans (bad weather) and ducks (good weather). " The savage utters and represents in his rites his will to live, his intense desire to live ; but it is desire and will and longing, not certainty and satisfaction that he utters " (Jane Harrison). Hence the contest becomes an appropriate symbol. The origins of many things become lost from view in course of time, and when we witness a test match or a Noel Coward revue, their primitive religious significance certainly does not leap to the eye.

The " Bacchæ " was Euripides's swan-song and was produced after his death. It may be held to contain the evening of his thought, but how it can be imagined to hold a recantation of his earlier agnostic questionings I cannot conceive. Professor Gilbert Murray says : " The reader . . . will be startled to find how close this drama, apparently so wild and imaginative, has kept to the ancient rite. The regular year-sequence is just clothed in sufficient myth to make it a story." The god Dionysus comes to his own land and is rejected by his kinsman, King Pentheus, who binds and imprisons him. The women watching for the appearance of the god from the stable in which he was imprisoned, and his triumphant resurrection, are forcible reminders of the way in which man has always fashioned his deity in the image of the harvest and the vintage—bread and wine. The risen god entices Pentheus to join in his rites, disguised in his mother's clothes. (Some may read the idea of mother fixation here.) He is torn into fragments by the Mænads, and his mother, maddened by the god, returns in triumph with her son's head, which she has taken for a lion's. (Some also may read here the symbol of the all-powerful mother, destroying that to which she has given birth.) And then the god restores the survivors to their senses and to misery.

Gilbert Murray says: "This bewildering shift of sympathy (from Dionysus to Pentheus and his mother) is common in Euripides. Oppression generates revenge, and the revenge becomes more horrible than the original oppression. In these plays the poet offers no solution. He gives us only the bitterness of life and the unspoken ' tears that are in things '."

Why should we speculate as to whether Euripides approved or disapproved of either Dionysus or Pentheus ? Nature is both fertile and cruel, he seems to say, and who shall gainsay him ?

This creation of the god by the rite was forcibly impressed on my mind when I saw a performance of the " Bacchæ " at Cambridge. For looking back at the succession of Greek plays since one was an undergraduate, one can realize how from the recurrent rite the idea of an immortal god arose in the minds of the Greeks. Here it was made manifest before the eyes—in the stalls the ageing audience, on the stage eternal youth.

If we climb a little higher up the steep slope of the Acropolis from the theatre of Dionysus we shall find the Temple of Æsculapius which, as we have seen, illustrates how another insistent fear of man has made another god—not the dread of starvation, but the dread of disease. The cult of Æsculapius was of comparatively late origin and first came into prominence in historical times. In the epic of heroic times he figures as a skilled physician. Homer makes him a pupil of Cheiron the Centaur.

A still earlier example of the physician being first looked upon as a demigod and finally as a god was Imhotep, who lived in Egypt about 2900 B.C. but who did not attain complete apotheosis until 525 B.C. In his cult, too, temple sleep was used, and indeed the whole ritual so closely resembled that in Æsculapian temples that it is difficult to resist the conclusion, considering how much the Greeks borrowed from Egypt, that the cult of Æsculapius was also borrowed. Imhotep was a real person, Æsculapius probably a mythical being. It would be in accordance with Greek methods if the rite preceded the god ; the desire for health becoming personified in a god later, whereas in Egypt the practices of an actual physician attained such sanctity as to make their inventor regarded as divine long afterwards. It is a further hint as to the close resemblance between these cults that when Greeks ruled Egypt in the days of the Ptolemies temples of Imhotep became temples of Æsculapius. But for further information I must refer you to the late Dr. J. B. Hurry's interesting book on Imhotep.

Now I come to another aspect of the god-making impulse, and I find it at Delphi. But it is not of the Delphic oracle, that token of man's insistent desire to question the future, that I am going to refer, but to a token of man's craving for physical security. Any of you who have visited Delphi will remember the scene : under the snowy heights of Parnassus stand the two shining cliffs which meet above the clear Castalian spring. As the road winds past the spring it is overshadowed by the giant plane tree, the descendant of that said to have been planted by Agamemnon. Below stand the ruins of the home of the Delphic Amphictony, the first attempt at a League of Nations. But our steps must lie in the other direction, up the hill, along the Sacred Way, past the temple of the Oracle, past the Treasury of Marathon to a spot where in 1913 was found an object of rough limestone shaped like half an egg. The Greeks believed that Delphi was the centre of the earth, and this object represented its omphalos or navel. It was pierced by a square hole, from which sprang the sky pillar. Primitive man was haunted by the fear that the inverted bowl of the sky would fall upon him. When Horace proclaimed, "Let justice be done, though the heavens fall," he spoke in a more sceptical age, but he spoke the language of an evolving moral consciousness. Not for him the crude superstition of a capricious, vindictive God who crushed the heavens down on the unfortunate creatures he had made. There was something higher than such a God, something more abstract, the conception of justice. To that and not to divine caprice he did homage. Fairy tales often embody primitive beliefs, and when Mr. A. B. Cook was studying the significance of this sky pillar he was reminded by his daughter how Cocky-Locky and Henny-Penny went to tell the King the sky was falling. The practical primitive, not trusting to the King's' power and fearing the falling of the roof of the sky, " proceeded to shore it up—first by a great central pillar, or terminal, rising from the omphalos, and next by two side pillars, east and west. The terminal was probably a roof tree to begin with, and then when the forest was left behind it became a sky-pillar joining earth and heaven. From the two side props sprang all the twin sun-gods, the Dioscuri and the like." Thus the twin gods, Castor and Pollux, who rescued the Romans from being over-whelmed by the Etruscans, were born of the fear that the heavens might fall. In their new security from their secular enemy it is not surprising that the Romans symbolized their deliverance as due to the twin gods who kept the heavens in place. As we stand in the Roman Forum to-day and see of all the magnificent temple of Castor and Pollux just three columns remaining, crowned by their entablature, we can imagine the ghost of an ancient Roman saying : " See, still they stand—the sky pillar and its twin supports—Rome is still immortal."

The triumphal arch has much the same significance, for its curve " represented the heavenly vault, and the triumphing general whose statue stood upon it was viewed as an embodiment of the sky god uplifted on his mimic sky ". The hero raised to the sky as a god. " The Marble Arch and the Arc de Triomphe, architecturally so insignificant, put on a new meaning " ; they are the outcome of a deep-rooted religious conviction, the significance of which has dwindled until, as Mr. Cook observes, " the monument that once stood for apotheosis now merely marks a stage for the motor omnibus." But was it, I wonder, an unconscious reversion to this ancient tradition that caused France to select the Arc de Triomphe as the burial place for her Unknown Warrior ?

But this is not the only example of the stone pillar as a god. We are so accustomed to the idea of Hermes as a swift messenger of Olympus that it is rather a shock to learn that in his original form he was a square pillar, later surmounted by a head. " In front of it was a hearth made of stone, with bronze lamps clamped to it by lead. Beside it an oracle was established. He who would consult the oracle comes at evening, burns incense on the hearth, lights the lamps, lays a coin on the altar to the right of the image, and whispers his question into the ear of the god. Then he stops his ears and quits the market place, and when he is gone outside a little way he uncovers his ears and whatever word he hears he takes for an oracle." No contrast could seem more complete than that between the square boundary stone and the winged messenger. What is the link between them. Miss Jane Harrison found it in Russia, where

255

the eastern Slavs used to burn the body of the dead man and place the ashes in an urn on a pillar or herm where the boundaries of two properties met. Now the name for grandfather and for boundary is the same in Russian. The offence of moving a neighbour's landmark is expressed in the phrase " beyond his grandfather ". The grandfather looked after the family during his life, he safeguarded its boundaries in death. His monument was at once tombstone and term. Such is the origin of terminal figures.

" Light begins to dawn. Hermes is at first just a Herm, a stone or pillar set up to commemorate the dead; into that pillar the mourner outpours, ' projects ' all his sorrow for the dead protector, all his passionate hope that the ghost will protect him still." When in the autumn he sows his seed he buries it in the ground as he buried his dead father or grandfather, and he believes that the dead man takes care of it . . . and sends it up to blossom in spring. . . . And more than this, in their lifetime a man went to his elders for advice—surely they will not fail him now. So at night he steals to the Herm and asks his question. The Herm is dumb, but the first chance word the man hears comes to him as an oracle from the dead. . . . But it is not only the seeds and the flocks that the dead ancestor must watch over. More important still, he is the guardian of the young, the children of his clan. . . . And finally when he is translated to Olympus he still watches over the infant gods, and Praxiteles so fashioned his image, Hermes carrying the child Dionysus. How exactly the leap to Olympus was accomplished we do not know. . . . The old boundary god, the steadfast Herm had been the medium of communication with the ghosts below ; it was natural that he should be the messenger of the gods above, but he must change his shape. His feet once rooted to the ground are freed and fitted with winged sandals, his magician's staff with its snakes he keeps, only now it has become a herald's staff, and he himself has shed his age and is a young man, " with the first down on his cheeks." It is as the messenger that modern art and literature remember Hermes, the messenger and herald :—

"New-lighted on a heaven-kissing hill."

This is Miss Harrison's interesting interpretation of the evolution of a boundary post into a messenger of the gods. It throws new light on the compact between Jacob and Laban. The Herm is the symbol of the divine right of property, of frontiers. It must date from the end of a period of nomadic wanderings, when men settled down to till their own land. The worship of the frontier post is also one of the latest manifestations of the god-making tendency in man. A nation prefers to govern itself badly rather than to be governed well by someone else. The native land begins to assume the features of a god. We say glibly that Germany wants this, Italy does that, and so on. What does it mean ? Very often merely that some individual or a small group seizes the ear of the public, generally by the aid of the press or wireless and forces his or their ideas upon them. No longer the worshipper whispers into the ear of the Herm ; the god shouts into the ear of the worshipper as he sits at breakfast. Irresistibly this recalls the hollow statue of the god into which the priest creeps and makes his own words into the divine utterance. And in many countries to-day the people seem actually to prefer a vicegerent of the national god in the flesh, and the dictator replaces democracy.

But the time has come for me to try and draw some general conclusions from these scattered instances of the deep-seated tendency of men to make gods. Dr. Charles Singer points out that each religious system in its day was an attempt to explain Man and the World and their relation to each other. Each system deals, too, with man's origin and his fate. " They have all sought to provide their followers with an explanation of the world in which they live. Such cosmologies were once the very bases of the appeal that these religions made to the rationalizing mind. Historically we now know that on another mental level such cosmologies form an obstacle where once they were an aid.

In trying to formulate my conclusions it is necessary for me to make clear that I am only explaining the mechanisms by which it seems to me the expression of the religious impulse has developed. To explain such mechanisms historically does not explain either the origin or the destination of that impulse. I often smile at the complaint that science tries to " explain away " things. For it seems to me that the revelations of science only deepen the sense of mystery, replacing some childlike and inadequate interpretation by something which strains our utmost intelligence to grasp.

The development of the Atomic Theory from Dalton to Rutherford has already rendered it impossible " to make pictures with our senses in regions where the senses cannot enter ". One might say that even the electron has about the same relation to reality as a child's calculating board of marbles threaded on wires has to higher mathematics. This illustrates the view I advanced before ; the nearer we approach the concrete image the more we realize that it is merely the symbol of something beyond. If you will concede that point, I hope I can formulate my views without offence. I shall avail myself of some of the arguments and illustrations given by Miss Jane Harrison in her Epilegomena to the study of Greek Religion wherein she gathered together the fruits of her life work.

The religious impulse is primarily directed to the conservation of the common life, physical and spiritual. Religious rites are primarily of two kinds, expulsion and impulsion. Primitive man has, in order that he may live, the old dual task, to get rid of evil and to secure good. In the rite there is a certain tension either of remembrance or anticipation. At first there is no idea of a god in this, but the emotion aroused gradually leads on to representation. Primitive man figures to himself what he wants and he creates an image of it which is his god. " A god so projected *is* part of the worshipper and is felt and realized as such. The dancer in the sacred rite cannot be said to worship his god, he lives him, experiences him." We cannot say with certainty when severance took place, but " the process of personification led to severance, and personification was undoubtedly helped by two things : (1) the existence of a leader to the band of worshippers ; (2) the making of puppets or images." We have seen how Dionysus was a deified form of successive leaders of the dances, and how Hermes arose from the boundary stone. At this stage he is more like a daimon, a kind of familiar spirit.

" The daimon is born of the rite, and with the rite that begat him he is doomed. The gradual dwindling and death of the rite is inevitable. Magic is found again and again to be a failure. . . . The rite fails, but the daimon projected from the rite remains. . . . The presentation, as it were, is cut loose. Out of this desolated, dehumanized daimon bit by bit develops the god. He is segregated aloof from the worshipper, but he is made in the image of that worshipper, so must be approached by human means, known by experience to be valid with other human beings, and such are prayer, praise, and sacrifice. . . . This segregation of the image from the imagination that begot it . . . in most religions develops into a doctrine and even hardens into something of a dogma. Man utterly forgets that his gods are man-begotten and he stresses the self that separates himself from his own image and presentation. This is very notable in Greek religion."

At this stage we recall the Olympian type of gods who " reflect the passions of their worshippers and not infrequently lag behind them in morality ". And as the god becomes separated from man, the rites out of which he arose assume new forms. The fertility dance becomes the drama, and the Temple of Æsculapius becomes the Hospital and Medical School.

For the purpose of refuge and strength " a god of the Olympian type serves best. A god of the daimon type is too near, too intimate for relief ". But with the advance of thought destructive criticism comes into play. The origin of the god is inquired into ; he is found inadequate. It is realized again that the god is the expression of the soul's sincere desire, and the idea of Immanence takes shape. This is at least as old as St. Augustine, yet it lies at the root of Modernism. The god within us assumes new importance. The desire expressed first as rite, then as daimon, and then as Olympian deity is recognized more accurately for what it is. But this is not enough—it does not explain why man should desire to rise. It does not explain why, biologically speaking, every scrap of protoplasm is out to develop itself to the utmost, or why in the interests of the community it may actually desire to sacrifice itself. The problem is to harmonize the god within and the god above, to reconcile immanence and tran- scendence. On this point I may refer you to a very interesting article on Theism and Pantheism by Professor Alexander in the *Hibbert Journal* for January, 1927. I can only quote a few salient sentences. " Whereas upon the current notions man being less than God may need for his religious satisfaction a man in whom God is embodied, for the forward view man's life is preparatory to the outgrowth of the divine quality. Every man is in this notion prophetic of deity. . . . God is not the already perfect being who for the benefit of imperfect man takes human shape, but is himself in the making, and his divine quality or deity a stage in time beyond the human quality. And as the root and leaves and sap of the plant feeds its flower, so the whole world, as so far unrolled in the process of time, flowers into deity. . . . God's deity is thus the new quality of the universe which emerges in its forward movement in time." He claims that a God thus conceived would be consistent with the nature of the world as we know it in the guise it presents to the other sciences. I must say that it appeals to my biological training, and it renders intelligible the stages of god- making I have described. These stages represent not

260

error but imperfect apprehension of the truth, adapted to the intelligence of the age in which they occurred. That the stage we have reached represents the final one is, by all analogy and all history, highly improbable. Theology should be at least as capable of development and expansion as physics. The difficulty is that so many men desire to be static, just because they demand the immediate satisfaction that would come from complete explanation. Desiring certainty they grasp at a manifestly inadequate explanation and proclaim that it is the whole truth. But truth goes marching on.

> We are the Pilgrims, Master ; we shall go
> Always a little farther.

THE LAND OF ST. FRANCIS

4th October, 1926.

There is significance in the very spontaneity of the celebration of the seventh century of St. Francis's death. To some he is the rediscoverer of the spirit of Christianity, to some he represents an almost pantheistic delight in the world of nature, to others, as to Renan, he is the father of Italian art. Certainly his life inspired Giotto to many of his happiest efforts.

It is true that a more humanitarian attitude had begun to prevail even before his time ; St. Bartholomew's Hospital was already more than fifty years old when he was born. But it was in St. Francis that this spirit found its most complete expression. It is perhaps just because his life was a protest against formalism and materialism that his influence is so strong to-day, because it is so much needed.

Wilfred Trotter has said : "Let a man beware of disciples." It is doubtful how far Plato modified the teaching of Socrates ; some would point to a still more exalted example of a Master's teaching being altered by a disciple. Certain it is that even in St. Francis's lifetime men like Elias and Leo so profoundly altered the Order he founded that he could no longer find a place within its ranks. It is the common fate of all great teachers. Soon after his death they heaped three churches, one over the other, on top of his body, as if determined that his spirit should no longer move among men. The small home in which he lived and worked, the Portiuncula, is emblazoned with inappropriate frescoes and enclosed in the enormous church of Santa Maria degli Angeli. But all in vain ; for the man was greater than any building.

Not that the churches of San Francesco are not beautiful. The crypt wherein his body lies may be pretentious with its nineteenth century restorations, but the lower and upper churches have been designed to form a striking and appropriate contrast. The lower church is filled with a dim solemnity, its arches are low, its structure massive. The upper church is full of light and space ; its arches soar, its spirit is joyous. The same contrast is expressed in the frescoes, which are dignified in the lower church, full of sunshine in the upper. Of the latter, St. Francis preaching to the birds is the best known and most favourite example, showing Giotto at his best.

Umbria has been called the land of poverty and peace. Even to-day industrialism has only faintly touched its fringe, without alleviating its poverty or disturbing its peace very much. Standing on the terrace at Perugia where once stood the papal fortress, one sees the Umbrian valley crowned by its ring of hill towns, very much as they appeared in his day. There is the Roman bridge across the Tiber over which he walked, there springs the River Clitumnus out of the rock, clear and cool as when its praises were sung by Roman poets. There stand Trevi, Spello, Spoleto that repulsed Hannibal, Montefalco, and many others. But most of all does Assisi, " a rose red city, half as old as time," focus the attention. And it is chiefly because of St. Francis that the eye seeks it out. Every hour that splendid vista changes with the changing light. But it is most beautiful when the sun sinks behind the hills and the valley is filled with a luminous violet haze. And as the daylight fades and the lights sparkle on each hill town there forms a picture that does not soon fade from the memory.

This view is the best initiation to the land of St. Francis, the land whence came the light that dispelled the Dark Ages. Goethe visited the Temple of Minerva at Assisi, and having seen it walked down the hill again without turning his steps towards San Francesco. This gives a measure of the difference between his time and ours ; to-day such indifference is unthinkable.

But though Assisi is the centre of interest in this fascinating country, the memory of St. Francis will impel the traveller to climb up into the mountain fastnesses to which he at times retired for rest. One such is the Carceri, nestling in a cleft of Mount Subasio. Twenty years ago one might see a shepherd, clad in sheepskins, standing on the sky-line as one toiled up to the little monastery in the woods. The gate was opened by a jolly old custodian, like Simon the Cellarer, who refreshed the heated traveller with a draught of wine cooled in the depths of the monastery well. Here one could see the very haunts of St. Francis and walk in his wooded garden. To-day the ascent is easier, thanks to the road made by the Austrian prisoners of war. The wild-looking shepherds have vanished and Simon is gathered to his fathers, but the tiny monastery is the same as ever. The birds still sing in the garden of St. Francis, finding sanctuary here from the " sportsmen " who, fearfully and wonderfully clad, sally forth every week to kill even sparrows elsewhere in Italy.

To-day Assisi will be thronged with pilgrims ; they will crowd into the garden of thornless roses at the Portiuncula, and then climb the hill to San Francesco, which glows as it has glowed for nigh on seven hundred years with the very beginnings of that art which has made Italy famous throughout the world. Their motives may be mixed and various, but if we would seek an explanation of why to-day the thoughts of so many turn to the " Poverello " of Assisi we may find it in these words : " Such an appeal as that of St. Francis can never be understood unless it is remembered how there were and there are on his side the hidden longings and the lost dreams of mankind and all its hopes so long deferred."

ON EVOLUTION IN ITALIAN ART

Every great epoch in art runs its course in an astonishingly short time. When Botticelli was born in 1447 Fra Angelico was still actively painting ; when he died in 1510 Raphael and Titian were established masters. Indeed, except for the earlier group of primitives, his sixty years of life overlapped those of all the great masters of Italian painting. The great period of Greek Art and the Elizabethan drama had even a shorter life. Men like Lyly and Greene and Nash evolved the drama from the Miracle Play and the Morality. Their importance, to quote Addington Symonds, " consists in their having contributed to the formation of Marlowe's dramatic style. It was he who irrevocably decided the destinies of the romantic drama ; and the whole subsequent evolution of that species, including Shakespeare's work, can be regarded as the expansion, rectification, and artistic ennoblement of the type fixed by Marlowe's epoch-making tragedies. In very little more than fifty years from the publication of Tamburlaine, our drama had run its course of unparalleled energy and splendour." First the development of the form and technique, then the full-blown flower and then its decay in baroque extravagance. It is only necessary to mention the so-called Throne of Aphrodite now in the Baths of Diocletian, the Hermes at Olympia and the Laocoon in the Vatican to show that exactly the same sequence occurred in Greek sculpture. Spring, summer, and autumn follow as inevitably as in the seasons of the year.

All this is so well recognized as to be hardly worth insisting on. There is, however, another less well recognized biological law, which is in apparent contradiction with

265

this. Once life has started it inevitably runs its course—true ; but in lowly organisms we meet with a phase of suspended animation when conditions are unfavourable, the phase of encystment, which may be indefinitely prolonged, and emergence from which is followed by an active phase of rejuvenescence. And I find in Byzantine art the parallel to this state of suspended animation, since for about a thousand years it persisted with only minor changes as displayed in mosaic. This is broadly true, for despite the differences between the glowing splendours of the Capella Palatina at Palermo, the delicate pictures in the Convent of Daphni, and the tender tones of Galla Placidia's Mausoleum at Ravenna, where the artificer worked intently on his representation of the Good Shepherd while the world as he knew it was falling to pieces, there is no obvious development until we reach the Kariyeh Mosque in Constantinople where the mosaics are coming to life in spiritual kinship with Giotto's frescoes. The crude frescoes in the Catacombs have always excited interest, but for me their chief interest is the extraordinary decadence they show when compared with the exquisite decoration of Augustan houses. By the time of Constantine all artistic impulse seems to have died down ; his very Arch is a fraud, stolen from the Arch of Trajan and clumsily brought up-to-date. But when he moved his capital to the Bosphorus a new art arose, best known in mosaic, but assuming many other forms such as enamels and carvings in ivory. To-day we are realizing how much of this art came from Persia to blend with what remained from the Greek. A revenge for Marathon indeed ! When most of Europe was ravaged by barbarian hordes the lamp of learning and of art still went on flickering at Constantinople, and when the Middle Ages began to develop a new culture it was from Constantinople that the germ of pictorial art came. That it came through a criminal act is beside the mark now. For in 1204 the Crusaders, balked of their legitimate prey, sacked Constantinople, chiefly at the instance of Venice. We prefer to close our eyes to that fact, and to forget that all the Crusades except the first were preposterous failures. If we did not, we should be less ready to use a term that really covered itself with disgrace. But of all the episodes that disgraced the Crusades none was so shameful as this sack of Constantinople. It enriched unscrupulous Venice, to be sure, but that was hardly the purpose for which the Crusades were undertaken. But it fatally weakened the extreme outpost against the Turk, who later overwhelmed it and advanced even to the walls of Vienna.

This earlier sack of Constantinople brought into Italy a number of Greek painters and pictures. The encysted life took on a fresh growth in its new environment. Setting aside Cimabue, if there ever was " sich a person ", Duccio in Siena and Giotto in Florence transformed the old Byzantine mode into something new and living. The stiff hieratic forms lived and moved and had their being. We must not forget the influence of St. Francis of Assisi in this proto-Renaissance, if such a hybrid term may be permitted. As Clutton-Brock says : " When the baleful and inhuman Gods of Byzantine art grew more anthropomorphic, it may well have been due to his influence. He induced men to take an interest in the beauty of the visible world, which had previously been considered, perhaps not quite explicitly, as a snare of the devil." Certain it is, at any rate, that in the Church at Assisi, erected over his grave, we find the finest examples of this early vital art. But by the middle of the fourteenth century this impulse in its turn seems to have died down, and there is a gap of more than fifty years before the new and stronger growth began. This is a point which is often overlooked, and is the more remarkable when we remember its rapid and vehement development when it had once started. And here we encounter a curious result of political jealousy. Siena and Florence were rivals, and Duccio started the Sienese School just before the Florentine School began to blossom. Proud of their priority, the Sienese School maintained their style as untouched as possible, and steadfastly refused to accept any of the innovations that radiated from Florence. For two hundred years after Duccio the Sienese changed their style as little as possible. Towards the end of that time it was clear that they were being deliberately archaic ; Francesco di Giorgio was contemporary with Raphael, yet he affected the primitive manner. Charmingly decorative, he was yet as deliberately out of touch with the art of his time as our pre-Raphaelites were with that of theirs. This resistance to progress finally met with the inevitable fate of all failure in adaptation. The Sienese people wearied of this local brand of art and Sodoma was imported and given important commissions. His new emotional way of painting captivated them, and the Sienese School came to an end. Byzantine art could remain static because the conditions were static, but Italy in the sixteenth century was changing rapidly, and those changes in the end swept away resistance as the incoming tide sweeps away castles in the sand.

Florentine and Umbrian painting never tried to stand still. It was eager and experimental. The fall of Constantinople in 1453 enormously stimulated an interest in the Classics, and mythological subjects largely replaced sacred ones. The old gods came to life once more and inspired some of Botticelli's most beautiful pictures. The obsession of sin weakened and man's spirit rose. Even in sacred pictures the note changed ; the emphasis was different. You can trace it in the representations of the Madonna. The early pictures follow the stiff, hieratic tradition and the next lay stress on the virginity ; but now the emphasis is laid on maternity. This, they seem to say, is akin to the miracle that may happen in any home. Compare Raphael's Madonnas with Lippo Lippi's if you doubt this. Of Raphael it may be said that it is necessary to pass through three phases to appreciate him. At first one accepts him on tradition as a very great painter, and then passes on to agree with those who consider that he painted extremely well in the manner in which any commonplace individual would like to paint. Only after passing through this stage can one realize the greatness of the man. True he fixed the style, and his followers killed it, but we must forget the imitators and realize his matchless construction and design, his flowing rhythms and his soaring imagination. If we find him conventional, we must remember that he created the convention.

Whether the Crusaders' sack of Constantinople initiated the rise of Italian painting or no, the sack of Rome in 1527 by Charles V indubitably ended it. Only in remote Venice did it linger on. Titian, Palma Vecchio, and Giorgione started together, and it is usually thought that the last-named was the dominant influence at first. To Giorgione the formation of their distinctive style is usually attributed. It is at any rate probable that he introduced the psychological note which Titian elaborated. This is well seen in " The Tempest ". Art critics complain that this picture has no central point of interest. But it portrays tempest without and tempest within, and the central point is the flash of lightning that divides the picture obliquely, separating the figure of the man from that of the woman and child. The parable is clear, and is emphasized by the two broken columns on the fountain. Titian survived Giorgione by nearly half a century, and developed their methods to great heights of glowing colour and emotional significance. It is interesting to find that in a letter to Philip II of Spain he spoke of being engaged on " two new poesies ". Clearly, then, we are justified in assuming that his pictures were intended to express something more than merely " significant form ", which some modern critics assure us is all that we should look for. He continued to paint until his hundredth year, though towards the end his pictures acquired a grimness that is foreign to the rest. There is a similar macabre note in Franz Hal's last picture, now hanging where he died in Haarlem.

After Titian, Venetian art still continued, though it gradually changed its form as Venice came to merit the description of " the Monte Carlo of its day ". But in the rest of Italy art died with Michael Angelo, who, indeed, despite his genius, was the father of the baroque. The Eclectic Schools of Rome and Bologna followed the method of compilation. They selected the colour of one master, the design of another, and the technique of a third, expecting in this way to resume the excellencies of all. Unfortunately they left out the essential ingredients— the genius that inspired each.

Is there not a similar danger to-day ? I was recently assured by a well-known critic that the principles of art were now known and scientifically defined. But genius is indefinable. There is a tendency to intellectualize all the arts and rigidly to exclude emotion. They must be made incomprehensible except to the expert. To the onlooker art is in a chaotic state, seeking its inspiration anywhere and everywhere except in the classic forms. Whether this is believed to mark the end of an epoch or the dawn of a new one depends on the temperament, and largely on the age of the individual. I would how-ever suggest that as history records periods of artistic decadence, I may be right in my feeling that we are passing through such a one now. Yet however much my æsthetic susceptibilities may be outraged by the art of to-day, I am willing to hope that out of the present chaos a new art may still be born. The horizon of man's mind has widened enormously, not only by the material achievements of science but also by the stimulus it is affording to his imagination. After all hope is of things as yet unseen.

THE PLAGUE IN ENGLAND

The plague is a disease which has been known under several names—the black death, the pest, the botch, the Levantine or bubonic plague. How dire were its onslaughts is hinted by the significant fact that it has so often been simply termed *the* plague. Of all the specific fevers it was the most fatal. In one epidemic at Baghdad 55 per cent of the cases died, and in the Volga epidemic of 1879, 90 per cent, some villages being literally exterminated. At Eyam, in Derbyshire, 74 per cent of the entire population perished.

The first great outbreak of undoubted plague was in the reign of Justinian, A.D. 542. There is a tradition of an epidemic in Libya in the third century B.C. or even earlier, and Aretaeus speaks of Βουβῶνες λοιμώδες. But the great plague of Athens, so vividly portrayed by Thucydides, appears not to have been bubonic, but scarlatina maligna; while that at the time of Marcus Aurelius, described by Galen, seems to have been smallpox. You will find the story of this first epidemic of plague in Gibbon's stately page: "The fatal disease which depopulated the earth in the time of Justinian and his successors first appeared in the neighbourhood of Pelusium, between the Sorbonian bog and the eastern channel of the Nile. From thence, tracing as it were a double path, it spread to the east, over Syria, Persia, and the Indies, and penetrated to the west along the coast of Africa and over the continent of Europe. . . . The infection was sometimes announced by the visions of a distempered fancy, and the victim despaired as soon as he had heard the menace and felt the stroke of an invisible sceptre. But the greater number, in their beds, in the streets, in their usual occupations, were surprised by a slight fever

—so slight, indeed, that neither the pulse nor the colour of the patient gave any signs of the approaching danger." He then goes on to describe the symptoms of the disorder and its spread, and says : " In time its first malignity was abated and dispersed, the disease alternately languished and revived ; but it was not till the end of a calamitous period of fifty-two years that mankind recovered their health, or the air resumed its pure and salubrious quality. No facts have been preserved to sustain an account, or even a conjecture, of the numbers that perished in this extraordinary mortality. I only find that during three months, five, and at length ten thousand persons died each day at Constantinople ; that many cities of the East were left vacant, and that in several districts of Italy the harvest and vintage withered on the ground. The triple scourge of war, pestilence, and famine afflicted the subjects of Justinian ; and his reign is disgraced by a visible decrease of the human species, which has never been repaired in some of the fairest countries of the globe."

Probably this wave of pestilence broke upon our shore. Certainly during the next century there was a great epidemic in Britain and in Ireland. Bede tells us how it more than decimated the monks at Jarrow, until he, then a boy in the monastery, alone was left to help the abbot in the antiphonies and responses. The land relapsed into the barbarism from which it was slowly emerging, and even London was left deserted and in ruins. Whether this was due to war or pestilence may be open to doubt ; both views have been maintained. Sir Norman Moore pointed out to me the interesting fact that St. Paul's Cathedral is built right over what must have been one of the main thoroughfares of Roman London—Watling Street, which he maintained was hardly likely to have happened if the City had been continuously occupied. An early life of Fechin of Fore, an Irish saint who died in 664, states that a great plague was the cause of his death, of that of the two reigning kings, and of a vast number of people in the same year.

From this time till the Black Death of 1347 we have no clear history of bubonic plague in England. Famine pestilences abounded—two bad harvests consecutively were sufficient to exhaust the resources of the country, which had no adequate means of importation or storage. England was a byword for her famine-pestilences, as was Normandy for leprosy, and France for St. Anthony's fire or ergotism. Creighton points out the significant fact that this last disease, " which is the truest index of an inferior diet . . . had little or no place in our annals of sickness." It shows at least that the peasantry were not dependent on the bad rye-bread which seems to have been the staple diet of feudal Europe.

The Black Death of 1347-9 was the most fearful epidemic of bubonic plague which this country has known. Its very name, though of later date, suggests its virulence, for the hæmorrhages under the skin are only seen in the most malignant types of the disease. Another symptom was severe hæmorrhage from the lungs, which, in most epidemics a rare complication, was here very common.

Arising in the Far East, the pestilence poured into Europe by the usual trade routes—Baghdad, the Crimea, Aden, and Alexandria. At Caffe, in the Crimea, the Tartars were besieging the Genoese settlement, when the Black Death broke out among the assailants. With brutal cunning they, " by the aid of the engines of war, projected the bodies of the dead over the walls into the city," spreading the disease so rapidly as almost to exterminate the garrison. It reached Italy early in 1348 through Genoa and Venice. Of its ravages in Florence a vivid and truthful picture is to be found in Bocaccio : Petrarch's Laura died of the plague at Avignon. Rolling through France, the wave of pestilence seems to have divided, one going to Normandy, the other eastward to Calais. It was the western wave which broke on our shore first, reaching Weymouth in August, and spreading over the western counties before the end of the year. At Bristol, says Knighton, " died, suddenly overwhelmed by

273   T

death, almost the whole strength of the town, for few were sick more than three days, or two days, or even half a day." The contagion spread so rapidly throughout the land, that to follow its course accurately is impossible. London was reached, from one source or another, some time in the month of October. The mortality was so severe that new burial-grounds had to be opened ; one on the site of the Minories ; another in West Smithfield, between the gates of St. Bartholomew's Hospital and St. John's Gate, which is still standing in St. John's Lane ; the third on the site of the Charterhouse. Oxford suffered terribly ; here we are told, on the authority of a contemporary Chancellor of the University, there were 30,000 scholars assembled. " The school doors were shut, colleges and halls relinquished, and none scarce left to keep possession, or to make up a competent number to bury the dead " (Wood). The plague pit was dug, according to Thorold Rogers, in some part of New College garden. Nor was East Anglia less afflicted. Dr. Jessopp estimates that during the year ending March, 1350, more than half of its population had been swept away, but the basis of his calculations has been disputed. At Cambridge the plague pit was probably opposite St. John's College. " When the foundations of the new Divinity School were being laid," says Thorold Rogers, " I saw that the ground was full of skeletons, thrown in without any attempt at order, and I divined that this must have been a Cambridge plague pit." Dr. Jessopp extracts an interesting point from the Court Rolls. " On 28th of April, 1349, a dispute was set down to be adjudicated upon by the steward and a jury of the homage. It was a dispute between a husband and wife on a question of dower. . . . The dispute was never settled. Before the day of hearing came on *every one* of the wife's witnesses was dead, and her husband was dead too." A pilgrim from Spain told a tale even more startling. " After supping with his host (who with his two daughters and one servant had alone so far survived of his entire family, and who was not then conscious of any sickness upon him) he settled with him for his entertainment, intending to start on his journey at daybreak, and went to bed. Next morning, rising and wanting something from those with whom they had supped, the travellers could make no one hear. They then learnt, from an old woman they found in bed, that the host, his two daughters, and the servant had died in the night. On hearing this the pilgrims made all haste to leave the place " (Gasquet).

Well might the people have said, " The Angel of Death is abroad in the land ; you can almost hear the beating of his wings." England was left desolate and silent ; memorials of that calamity are still seen in the architecture of the land, in noble works never finished, or completed in a later style. For instance, Winchelsea Church, and the western towers of St. Nicholas, Yarmouth, have remained unfinished ever since those days. War with France was suspended for sixteen years. The poor were generally most affected. " And no wonder," writes Professor Thorold Rogers, " living as the peasantry did in close unclean huts, with no rooms above ground, without windows, artificial light, soap, linen ; ignorant of certain vegetables, constrained to live half the year on salt meat." But the educated classes did not escape, the mortality among the clergy being very severe. There was a great dearth of students at the Universities, and from the King's address to the bishops we learn that Oxford, once the home of learning, had become " like a worthless fig tree without fruit ". Half the entire population had perished, and the social effects were profound. As we look out to-day across the rural landscape it is interesting to remember that the hedges which are so conspicuous a feature originated at that date, the tenancies having to be split up into fields to make farming a success. For labourers were hard to seek, they were wandering off in search of better conditions, and the restrictions laid on them by the Statute of Labourers were inadequate to check them.

There is an amusing example of the old proverb, " The devil was sick, the devil a monk would be," in the fact that during the Black Death the dice manufacturers found that to do any business they must convert their dice into paternosters. But no sooner had the scourge passed away than there was an instance of Niebuhr's aphorism : " Almost all great epochs of moral degradation are connected with great epidemics." Piers Plowman tells us of the great declension of morals " sithen the pestilence ". Cardinal Gasquet, a scholarly writer on the Black Death, said in 1893 : " It is a well ascertained fact, strange though it may seem, that men are not as a rule made better by great and universal visitations of Divine Providence. It has been noticed that this is the evident result of all such scourges ; or, as Procopius puts it, speaking of the great plague in the reign of the Emperor Justinian, ' Whether by chance or Providential design it strictly spared the most wicked.' So in this visitation, from Italy to England, the universal testimony of those who lived through it is that ' It seemed to rouse up the worst passions of the human heart and to dull the spiritual senses of the soul.' "

From the time of the Black Death till the great plague of 1665 the disease seems to have been periodically epidemic in Britain ; always smouldering, it occasionally burst into conflagrations throughout the fifteenth and sixteenth centuries. The plague of 1464 was said to have been foretold. " A boy at Cambridge, while walking in the lane between King's College and the adjoining building of Clare and Trinity Halls, met an old man with a long beard, who addressed him thus : ' Go now and tell to anyone that within these two years there will be such pestilence and famine and slaughter of men as no one living has seen.' Having said this he disappeared." It says something for the growth of scientific scepticism that doubts were at once cast on this story.

The sweating sickness, of which we hear a good deal in the years following the battle of Bosworth, can be clearly differentiated from plague, and was very probably a severe type of influenza. We hear the last of it in this form in 1551. Whereas plague always started with the poorer classes—so much so, indeed, that it was commonly called the " poor's plague "—the sweating sickness was most prevalent among the better classes ; nor, as a rule, did these diseases appear in the same year. The great advances which this country made in Tudor times naturally led to more stringent regulations for the check of plague, but for a long time apparently without effect. Anthony Wood records thirty outbreaks of plague in Oxford during the sixteenth century, " which led to great decline in the learning and *morale* of the place," " occasioned, as 'twas thought," says Wood, " by the overflowing of the waters, and the want of a quick passage for them from the ground : also by the lying of many scholars in one room or dormitory in almost every hall, which occasioned nasty air and smells, and consequently diseases."

The epidemic of 1563 largely affected the neighbour-hood of St. Bartholomew's Hospital. " The worst locality," says Dr. Jones in his *Dyall of Agues*, " was St. Sepulchre's parish, by reason of so many fruiterers, poor people, and stinking lanes, as Turn-again Lane, Sea-coal Lane," etc. Turn-again Lane owed its name to the fact that it ran straight down to the Fleet ditch, from which there was no other method of return. The Fleet ditch, which ran outside the western wall of the city, along what is now Farringdon Street, entered the Thames at Blackfriars. Its filthy condition was clearly believed to play a part in the epidemic of 1593, and a memorial was prepared to get it stopped up ; it was shown to have been in the centre of the most infected district, and it was urged that " it is no material defence for the city, and half the ditch has been stopped these many years ".

London had, in fact, long outgrown its primitive walls, and the sanitarians of Tudor times strenuously opposed its further extension. From the time of Richard I to Henry VII it was a medieval walled city, with a population of from forty to fifty thousand. Outside the walls were a few parishes, and on the west a wide thinly populated suburb, formed in 1393 into the Ward of

Farringdon Without, which reached to Holborn Bars and Temple Bar. This outlying district had similar privileges to the City, and was referred to as the Liberties. The City walls had Ludgate and Newgate on the west, and turning just south of St. Bartholomew's Hospital, ran along the route now indicated by London Wall ; and its northern gates were Aldersgate, the small Cripplegate, Moorgate, and Bishopsgate. On the east was Aldgate and the small postern gate just by the Tower, where the wall terminated. Just outside Moorgate was the Moor—a great fen, the sanitary condition of which was a dangerous nuisance to the City. Its situation is still indicated in the name Moorfields.

Henry V was one of the first to show great care of the public health. Probably he remembered the Moor as a danger to be avoided after copious libations at the " Boar's Head," Eastcheap ; Mistress Quickly's sack had a way of obscuring the points of the compass in the royal mind. Be that as it may, one of his first cares was to attempt to drain the Moor, and have roads laid down over it to the neighbouring villages of Islington and Hackney. But it was not till the time of Henry VIII that regular sanitary measures were taken. A certain level of plague was tolerated, but as soon as the infection became hot the well-to-do fled to the country.

In 1543 the following rules were put into force : The sign of the cross was to be put on all infected houses, with the inscription " Lord have mercy upon us " ; convalescents were to carry a white rod for forty days after, to mark them ; all straw in their houses burnt, and all clothes " cured " ; beggars were to be kept out of churches, and dogs were to be kept indoors, as infection was believed to be carried in their hair. The streets and lanes were to be scavenged and flushed.

Elizabeth went further—infected houses were to be shut up for forty days, no swine were to be kept within the City walls, and Simon Kellwaye published (1593) a code of rules which should be observed by all inhabitants. The queen herself retired to Windsor

278

during epidemics, and protected herself thus : " A gallows was set up in the market-place of Windsor, to hang such as should come there from London." No false feminine weakness for Queen Bess !

By this time the Liberties were much more crowded than the City itself. Freed from many of the restraints there enforced, outside the walls was a maze of dark and tortuous alleys, a paradise of jerry-building. Thus the old city became encircled by a fringe of all that was foul and unwholesome, and it was clear that many epidemics started in these outlying noisome slums. Elizabeth made gallant attempts to stem the evil ; no new houses were to be built within three miles of the City walls, subletting was made a misdemeanour punishable by law, but all in vain. London has steadily gone on growing, according to some " a wen on the face of civilization ", and the end we see not yet. William Morris's—

" Dream of London, small and white and clean,
The clear Thames bordered by its gardens green."

seems more visionary than ever.

Elizabeth's efforts were so far unavailing, that some years after her death we find the City, formerly the residence of the better classes, falling into the fate of Canongate, Edinburgh ; its mansions turned into tenements, its gardens and churchyards built upon. Meanwhile the suburbs of Westminster, Lambeth, Newington, and Stepney began to rise into importance, the last being from the first and for many years a highly fashionable suburb—a description hardly applicable to the Stepney of to-day. The following approximate numbers will give an idea of the growth of London in Tudor and Stuart times. At the time of the Reformation the population was about 60,000 ; a few years after the accession of Elizabeth, 90,000 ; eight years before the Armada, 120,000, and five years after it 150,000. At her death in 1603 it numbered about a quarter of a million—that is to say, during her reign of forty-five years it increased two and a half times. In spite of the turmoil of the civil wars we find it has again nearly doubled itself in 1662, being nearly half a million.

The Stuart epoch is marked by three great outbursts of plague and its final extinction. These outbursts occurred in 1603, 1625, and 1665. The epidemic of 1636 did not affect London very greatly, and it is these three alone that I need stop to discuss.

The best account of the plague of 1603 will be found in Thomas Dekker's book, *The Wonderful Yeare* 1603, *shewing London lying Sicke of the Plague.* Beginning in the suburb of Stepney, it spread over the City and Liberties, destroying between 19th March and 22nd December over 33,000 persons. It coincided with grave changes in the State : Queen Elizabeth died a fortnight after the outbreak, and James was to make a triumphal entry into London ; but a mightier monarch than he was already enthroned there, so the King stayed his course at Hatfield. " Every house," says Dekker, " lookt like St. Bartholomewe's Hospital," many that " would have been glad of a bed in an hospitall, and dying in the open fields, have been buried like dogs. . . . Never let any man aske me what became of our phisitions in this massacre —they hid their synodicall heads as well as the prowdest. Galen could do no more than Sir Giles Goosecap " ; and so on in the approved euphuistic mode. The flight to the country seems to have infected the neighbourhood of London more than was usual, Croydon and Enfield being particularly visited.

This plague was the occasion of one of the earliest English medical writings on the disease. Thomas Lodge, novelist, poet, and physician, published his treatise during the fatal year. His best remembered work will probably be not his medical writings, but his novel, *Euphues' Golden Legacy*—and that not because of its intrinsic merits, considerable though they be, but because his picture of Rosader and Rosalind and the forest wooing inspired Shakespeare to write his immortal *As you Like it*. How closely Shakespeare followed the story, and how enormously he lifted it by his genius will be seen by any who compare the two.

As for his treatise on the plague, we may note that he was one of the first to raise his voice against the barbarity of shutting up the infected houses in the way usually adopted. " For in truth it is a great amazement, and no lesse horror, to separate the child from the father and mother, the husband from his wife . . . For to speake the truth, one of the chiefest occasions of the deathe of sicke folke (besides the danger of their disease) is the fright and feare they conceive when they see themselves voyde of all succour and, as it were, ravished out of the hands of their parents and friends, and committed to the trust of strangers."

For several years after this there was a slight annual outbreak ; the playhouses were closed as soon as the mortality had reached a certain point, and reopened when the deaths fell to thirty a week. This gives us an idea of the way in which a certain endemic level of plague was tolerated and regarded as natural. But in 1625 the smouldering fires broke out again. The previous summer had been very hot and dry ; the winter was mild. On 25th February an exceptionally high tide flooded the riverside parts of London, filling Westminster Hall " full three feet in water all over ". Within a fortnight four deaths had occurred from plague, and the infection then spread in almost geometrical progression, culminating in 4,463 deaths in the week ending 18th August, and then, sinking down again, ended with the year. Allowing five days for incubation, and remembering that the third to the fifth day is the most commonly fatal, this places the deaths eight to ten days after the high tide, and we know from the bills of mortality the patients were buried within a fortnight of 25th February.

The total number of deaths in this epidemic was from forty to fifty thousand. The literature is not extensive. Almost the only utterance of at all a professional nature was from the pen of one Stephen Bredwell, of Oxford, who obtained the L.R.C.P. in 1594. This work I have not personally consulted for, according to Creighton, it is merely a shameless advertisement of " his 1*s*. powders and 2*s*. 6*d*. electuaries ". But Dekker again wrote on this epidemic—a fact I have not seen referred to in the literature of the subject ; his pamphlet is entitled *A Rod for Runawayes*, and is a castigation of the rich who sought refuge in flight, leaving the poor without a helper. This, in the then unorganized state of charity, was undoubtedly a serious matter. " How shall the lame and blinde and half-starved be fed ? They had wont to come to your gates ; alas ! they are barred against them." He further twits them with being unwelcome visitors : " The countrey-people stand there with halberds and pitch-forkes to keepe them out ; . . . if they spy but a footman (not having a russet suite on, their own countrey livery) they cry, Arme, charge their pike-staves before he comes near the length of a furlong ; and stopping their noses, make signes he must be gone, there is no roome for him to revell in, let him packe." He goes on to tell how some Londoners one Sunday morning essayed to walk across the fields to Kentish Town, but were seen by the worshippers in St. Pancras Church, who came out and drove them back to the town. He also remonstrates with those who conceal cases of plague to escape the restrictions, thinking to cheat the Almighty but, as he quaintly hath it, " His arithmetick brookes no crossing." Of the deserted state of London we get a vivid picture. " The walkes in Paul's are empty ; the streets in London too wide (here's no jostling)." George Wither also tells us in his wearisome poem on the subject—*Britain's Remembrancer*—

> " The walks are unfrequented, and the path
> Late trodden bare, a grassie carpet hath."

This latter carries his view that the epidemic is a Divine judgment to such particularity as to suggest it is due, among other factors, to—

> " Some imperfections
> In burgesses and their elections ! "

The plague of 1636 was not so extensive, nevertheless 10,400 deaths were reported. Heberden tells us it began in Whitechapel. And now with one final outburst the plague was to leave our shores for ever. Let me tell the story of its beginning in the language of its greatest observer—Thomas Sydenham.

"After an extremely cold winter, and after a dry frost that lasted without intermission until spring, and which then unexpectedly broke up in the early part of the year 1665, peripneumonies, quinsies, and all such inflammatory diseases suddenly caused a great mortality. At the same time an epidemic appeared, which was wholly different from the continued fevers that prevailed during the preceding constitution." As to the progress of the epidemic we must turn elsewhere, for Sydenham joined in the flight to the country. The College of Physicians appointed special physicians who agreed to stay in London and grapple with the plague ; among them we find Dr. Glisson, the distinguished Regius Professor of Physic at Cambridge, the well-known name of Paget, Dr. Wharton, Physician to St. Thomas's, Dr. Francis Bernard, afterwards Physician to St. Bartholomew's, and Dr. Hodges, who has left a good account in his *Loimologia* of the ordeal through which he passed. Another excellent description of the great plague is by Boghurst, the apothecary. This, the *Loimographia*, was left in MS. and first printed in 1894 by Dr. J. F. Payne. The most popular version is, of course, that by Defoe, one which will long live as literature, but untrustworthy for our purpose—for it is by no means the account of an eye-witness as it professes to be, Defoe being not more than five years old at the time. During the epidemic at Marseilles in 1720 there was a painful revival of interest in the subject, of which Defoe took advantage to secure many readers for his interesting novel. Such was the literary skill of Defoe that his fictions are clothed with what seems the sober veracity of history. It is untrustworthy, I say, for our purpose, for he undoubtedly follows Dekker's account of the earlier

283

plagues of the century, and applies it to 1665. As a matter of fact, those in authority had profited by experience, and good order appears to have been kept, the bills of mortality produced regularly, and an abundant supply kept in the markets. Creighton says that the dead were buried with full ceremony and in coffins till the heights of the epidemic in August and September. Then the bodies were brought in cartloads and thrown in ; in excavating for Broad Street Station, a stratum 4 feet down, and extending another 8 to 10 feet deep, was found which was full of uncoffined skeletons. Another plague pit was revealed as I saw myself when the foundations for the new General Post Office were dug in 1906. Still this probably did not occur to nearly the extent Defoe states, while it was common in the 1603 and 1625 epidemics. I shall venture to go beyond Creighton on this point, for at the height of the epidemic we read in Evelyn's Diary, under the date of 7th September : " I went all along the City from Kent Street to St. James's, a dismal passage, and dangerous to see so many coffins exposed in the streets, now thin of people." Moreover we have no proof that these pits do not date from 1603 or 1625.

The story of this epidemic is as an oft-told tale ; my repetition of it shall be brief. At the close of 1665, two or three persons died suddenly in one family at Westminster ; timorous neighbours moved into London and took the contagion with them. Long Acre was next attacked, and the infection spread through St. Giles's, down Holborn, and reached the City. Nevertheless the mortality did not attain double figures for the week till 23rd May, when fourteen died.

Then it began to increase rapidly, reaching 112 in the week ending 13th June. It was at the beginning of this week that Pepys notes : " This day, much against my will, I did in Drury Lane see two or three houses marked with a red cross upon the doors, and ' Lord have mercy ' writ there, which was a sad sight to me, being the first of the kind to my remembrance I ever saw. . . . Forced to buy some roll tobacco to smell and chew, which took away the apprehension." In passing I should remark that the eminent Diemerbroeck, who had experience of the plague in Holland in 1636, praised tobacco as a preventive. Hodges was uncertain as to its value ; personally, he tells us, he is its professed enemy, placing his reliance on sack.

Ten days later Pepys tells us : " It strucke me very deep this afternoon going with a hackney coach from my Lord Treasurer's down Holborne ; the coachman I found drive easily and easily, at last stood still, and came down hardly able to stand, and told me that he was suddenly strucke very sicke and almost blinde, he could not see."

The mortality was now spreading by leaps and bounds, being 1,082 in the week ending 18th July, 2,010 a fortnight later ; then increasing about 1,000 a week, it reached its height in the week ending 19th September. In that awful week 7,000 died in the City and Liberties, but if we include the suburbs Dr. Hodges tells us 12,000 was the total. By this time all who could fly had done so, the court had moved to Oxford, fires were burning in the streets, all was desolation. Says Pepys : " Grass grows all up and down White Hall Court, and nobody but poor wretches in the street." But the tide had turned, and next week saw a decrease of 2,000. October was ushered in with a weekly death-rate from plague of 4,300. Pepys writes under date of 7th October : " In the highway come close by the bearers with a corpse dead of the plague ; but Lord ! to see what custom is, that I am come to think almost nothing of it." A week later the deaths fell to one half, and by this time we hear " that in Westminster is never a physician, and but one apothecary left, all being dead ". The mortality remained at about a 1,000 per week till the middle of November, when it rapidly fell again, December seeing the average rate rather above 200. General confidence was restored, and the people flocked back to town, and displayed a foolhardiness only equalled by their former panic, actually, Hodges tells us, " using beds in which people had just died, before the rooms were even cleansed from the stench of the diseased." But the plague had spent its force, and many of those attacked recovered; and none too soon, for during that year 68,596 plague deaths were registered without counting the suburbs of Stepney, Lambeth, and Newington. I like to turn to the picture of sturdy old Dr. Hodges going about his avocation at a time when Pepys says: "This disease [is] making us more cruel to one another than if we were doggs." He rose early and took the quantity of a nutmeg of the anti-pestilential electuary; then spent two or three hours in a large room examining patients; then breakfast, followed by professional visits till dinner-time, putting some "proper thing" on the coals and keeping a lozenge in his mouth all the time; he naïvely tells us he kept his mind as composed as possible. He drank a glass of sack before dinner, and partook of easy and generous nourishment. He again visited till eight or nine at night, and "then concluded the evening at home by drinking to cheerfulness of my old favourite liquor, which encouraged sleep and easie breathing through the pores all night". During the whole time, he tells us, he felt ill but twice.

The plague lingered throughout 1666, causing in all 1,998 deaths, some 500 above its endemic level; in the first three weeks of December the deaths were two, four, and three, and never again rose from that point in London; a few deaths from it continued to appear in the bills of mortality till 1679, when the disease seems to have, as it were, finally flickered out. In the provinces, Cambridge, Eyam, and especially Colchester were severely affected in 1666; but that year saw the last of the disease in the provinces, except for a few cases at Peterborough in the first quarter of 1667.

The outbreak at Eyam is remembered not only for its severity, but still more for the story of the heroism displayed by all concerned. Eyam is a charming little village in Derbyshire between Buxton and Chatsworth. At that time it had quite a fair-sized population because

286

lead works were in operation there. During the outbreak of plague in London in 1665, some patterns of
cloth, or according to another story, the clothes of a
young man who had died of the disease were sent from
London to a tailor at Eyam. The tailor developed a
malignant form of plague and died in one day.

The rector of the parish, the Rev. William Mompesson
was a young man married only a few years ; his
wife was only twenty-seven and they had two small
children. They sent the children away and resolved to
stay at the post of duty. Mompesson wrote to London
for the most approved medicines and prescriptions ; he
also wrote to the Earl of Devonshire, as the title then was,
at Chatsworth, promising that his parishioners would
restrict themselves to their village provided that the Earl
would undertake that food, medicines, and other
necessities should be placed at certain appointed spots,
at regular times, upon the hills around, where the
villagers might come and take them, leaving payment
for them without holding any communication with the
bringers except by letters which could be placed upon
a stone and then fumigated before they were touched
by hand. The stone still stands and I have seen it on the
outskirts of the village ; it has a hollow at the top which
was kept filled with water, into which the money was
dropped. This engagement was duly observed throughout
the epidemic which lasted for seven months, and no cases
occurred outside the village.

Mr. Mompesson told his people that with the plague
once among them, it would be so unlikely that they should
not carry infection about with them that it would be
selfish cruelty to other places to try and escape thither,
thus spreading the danger. So rocky and wild was the
country around that, had they tried to escape, a regiment
of soldiers could not have prevented them. But of their
own free will they agreed to stay within the borders of
their own parish, and no one passed the boundary
throughout the whole of that terrible time.

The assembling of congregations had been thought

to spread the infection in London, so Mr. Mompesson thought it best to hold his services out of doors. In the middle of the village can be seen the dell he used for this purpose. On one side there is a sloping grass bank where his congregation sat, on the other almost perpendicular rocks. One of the rocks was hollow and could be entered from above, making a natural pulpit. The dell is so narrow that a voice could be clearly heard across it.

Day and night the rector and his wife were among the sick, feeding and nursing them ; but in spite of all their efforts only one-quarter of all the inhabitants survived. Mompesson buried those who died, not in his church-yard, for that might have perpetuated the infection, but on a heath high above the village. Week by week the congregation on the grassy slope of the dell grew smaller and smaller. Gradually they were passing to that heath on the hill.

Mompesson's health remained excellent throughout but, alas, his wife, exhausted by her efforts, took the plague and died. In the lull after the storm he wrote to his uncle as follows : " The condition of this place hath been so dreadful, that I persuade myself it exceedeth all history and example. I may truly say our town has become a Golgotha, a place of skulls. My ears have never heard such doleful lamentations, my nose never smelt such noisome smells, and my eyes never beheld such ghastly spectacles. Here have been seventy-six families visited within my parish out of which died 259 persons."

However now there were no fresh cases, and he burnt all woollen clothes lest the infection should linger in them. He lived many years after this terrible experience, indeed until 1708.

So virulent was the type of plague at Eyam that ninety-one years afterwards, when five working men were digging up land near the plague graves they came across some linen and all fell ill, though they had it buried it again immediately. Three of them died and no less than seventy persons in the parish were carried off. If that really was plague that was the last time that England saw it in epidemic form.

Plague so closely follows the type of diseases due to micro-organisms that although the bacillus was not found till 1894 by Kitasato, its existence had long been suspected—longer, in fact, than in any other disease, for Athanasius Kircher, in 1658, suggested that it was due to little worms so small and subtle that they escape every sense, and can only be detected by the most exquisite microscope. He believed these little worms to work their mischief by the elaboration of a poison. Here we have in brief the modern doctrine of micro-organisms and their toxins. But Kircher shows his modernity further by maintaining, in face of the prevailing belief, that a man cannot contract plague by imagination or fear alone, but that they only predispose " by condensation of spirits ". To-day we should say " by lowering of resistance " and be no wiser.

This view was of course too advanced for his age. Dr. Hodges, who, as we have seen, was one of the physicians appointed by the Royal College of Physicians to investigate the plague of 1665, confessed, with submission to so great a name, that he could never discover them, and humorously suggested that as the sky of Italy is brighter than in England, Kircher, who studied at Rome, was at an advantage.

The outbreak of plague in Hong Kong in 1896 which spread to India, Egypt, and Japan, and three years later to the Philippines and South America, enabled the disease to be studied by modern methods. It was noted that when a dead rat was found in a village, the inhabitants went away ; then it was discovered that the fleas which have fed on the blood of infected rodents, such as the large grey rat and the smaller black rat desert these animals after death and inoculate man when they bite him. Epidemics in rats invariably precede human epidemics. The infection is conveyed solely by means of fleas, and a case in man is not in itself infectious. Insanitary conditions are related to the occurrence of

U

plague only in so far as they favour infestation by rats. It will be seen therefore that the popular belief it was the Great Fire of London which exterminated plague in England represents only a small part of the truth ; certainly the destruction of so many old houses must have done away with many hiding places for rats, but that would not account for the almost simultaneous disappearance of epidemics from the provinces. It has been suggested that about that time the hardier brown rat, which is not infested by the special flea requisite, was introduced by ships and exterminated the black rat, previously so prevalent. It is interesting that, as I have stated, one epidemic started on the banks of the Fleet ditch and another after the flooding of Westminster Hall, for in each instance rats would probably be in the neighbourhood. In the case of Eyam infected fleas must have been present in the box of clothes. It is, however, difficult to imagine fleas living for ninety-one years in buried linen ! Within the last forty years insects have been shown to be the sole conveyors of four great scourges, plague, typhus, yellow fever, and malaria, which through the centuries have carried death and devastation before them. As Sir Arthur Shipley used to say it is the insects who contend with man for the mastery of the world.

THE EVOLUTION OF DEATH [1]

" Man alone among animals knows that he must die."
My subject is therefore perforce of interest to all, and I
hope to show that its scientific aspect is not altogether
gloomy. Fortunately the majority of men do not feel
with Dr. Johnson that " the whole of life is but keeping
away the thoughts of death ". As Milnes Marshall said :
" The problems of life are the most fascinating of all
scientific inquiries ; and surely death, the cessation of
life, must have something to teach us, must throw some
light on the nature of life itself. The beginnings of life
are at present hidden from us, the other end of the
series, the termination of life, we have daily opportunities
of studying. We are so accustomed to think of death as
the fate of all living things, that we forget that as all life
springs directly from pre-existing life, protoplasm really
is immortal." The flame is handed on from torch to
torch ; and though the torch may be extinguished, the
flame never is. How then did death arise ? Is it something
inherent in life itself or has it arisen for the benefit of the
race ? The question is too complex for us to begin its
study in the higher animals—we must turn to the simplest
forms of life.

The body, as we know, is composed of organs—the
stomach, the lungs, the heart, the brain, and so on.
Organs in their turn are composed of tissues—for instance,
connective nervous or muscular tissues. To analyse these
tissues further we require the aid of a microscope when
we find they are composed of what we call cells. This
is the unit of structure. If we compare a body with a
house, the organs are the rooms, the tissues the walls of
the rooms, and the cells are the bricks composing those

[1] An Address delivered at the Working Men's College.

walls. Each cell is typically composed of protoplasm, a complex jelly-like substance which is found in all living matter and it contains a denser portion, the nucleus, which is intimately bound up with the life of the cell. Frequently it is surrounded by a cell wall, and it may contain a vacuole, a clearer part containing a watery fluid or sap.

As we descend the scale of the animal kingdom we find increasing simplicity in the structure of the walls made by these bricks until at length we come to forms of life composed of only one cell—the Protozoa. In such animals it follows of necessity that all the functions of life must be discharged by that cell. Let us take as an example the amœba. Such an animal multiplies by simply dividing into two. The parent generation must thereby disappear but nothing has died : As Marshall neatly expresses it : " If the original amœba be called Tom and the products of the division Dick and Harry, the upshot of the process may be expressed by saying that Tom has disappeared without having died, while Dick and Harry have come into existence without having been born. Nothing has died, there is no corpse to bury, and our ordinary ideas with regard to individuality and identity fail altogether to afford answer to the question —Where is Tom at the end of the process ? "

Of course violent death may occur, but not natural death in such circumstances. From the first appearance of such animals right up to the present day there has been direct continuity of living matter. No such animal that meets a violent death can leave offspring, " For such offspring can only arise by the division of the living body of the parent "—no such animal " has ever left an ancestor by death ".

Going a little higher in the scale of life we find instances where such cells do not go about singly but cluster together in colonies. And it soon happens that the work done by each cell is not exactly the same. The principle of division of labour appears. In one striking example of a colony composed of 128 of such cells, the front ones chiefly look after the nourishment of the colony and only the hinder cells are capable of dividing to form new colonies. The front cells after a certain length of time die, but the hind cells do not—they are simply transformed by division into new individuals. In other words the front cells have relinquished their immortality and simply concern themselves with promoting the welfare of the colony.

Going still higher in the scale we find animals that are composed of many cells, and these cells differ both in structure and in function—instead of each cell doing everything for itself, different cells are told off to do one thing especially ; instead of each cell being self-supporting as it were, the whole labour of the body is divided up between the various cells. In such a case the power of forming new individuals is restricted to certain cells. These cells then are immortal in the same way as the amœba. They can be destroyed, but otherwise they do not die. They are derived from division of similar cells in preceding generations so that there has been direct continuity of living matter from generation to generation.

The many-celled animal is, of course, a much more efficient machine than the single-celled animal, but according to Weismann death is the penalty for possessing a body which must encounter wear and tear—the amœba, with its single cell, escapes the penalty because it only consists of the protoplasm used in the next generation. Every higher organism possesses some of this immortal protoplasm, but it must be handed on to the next generation if it is to be of any avail—it is the germ plasm.

Perhaps the most startling fact about protoplasm is the power it possesses of renewing its youth. This it may do in several ways. (1) Rest is a powerful restorative of protoplasm. Certain simple forms of life seem to lose all vitality for a time, and surround themselves by a thick capsule. But after a rest they come forth again with renewed energy. Just so a weaver by long habit ceases to notice the noise of the machinery, his nerve centres cease to respond to the oft-repeated stimulation. But let him take a holiday—on returning he is again conscious of the noise now that his senses have been freshened up. (2) Change of surroundings rejuvenates protoplasm. Some forms of life are unable to complete their life cycle unless they can do this. The fluke that inhabits the livers of sheep must at a certain stage migrate into a pond-snail—if it does not it simply dies. The protozoon that causes malaria must spend part of its life in man and part in the mosquito. This has been compared with the invigorating effects of a trip to the seaside, after which a man can return to his old occupations with increased advantage and renewed energy.

But despite these means of refreshment protoplasm unaided tends to senile decay. The Ribstone Pippin, once so famous among apples, is now almost extinct, for cuttings of it have hardly any vitality left. The Champion potato used to be immune to blight, and this made it the mainstay of the Irish peasantry in the potato famine of 1847. But this power of resisting blight it has now lost. Why should these special strains tend to die out, while others remain as vigorous as ever? Because they are propagated by slips, cuttings or grafts, and not from seeds. And the special feature of a seed is that it is the result of the union of two cells and not simply of the direct division of one cell. The key to the situation is here—the continued simple division of cells brings no fresh life, but the union of two cells having a nucleus and cell substance that were previously strangers to each other leads to complete rejuvenation of the protoplasm —in other words, fresh blood is infused into the firm of Nucleus, Protoplasm and Co., and the firm gets a new new lease of life.

Some experiments carried out by Maupas helped to establish these facts. He took a small one-celled Infusorian and followed its repeated subdivisions—between November, 1885, and March, 1886, this single cell had given rise to 215 generations. At the end of that time they all died, having shown signs of senile decay for some time previously. But if a single individual were removed and allowed to unite with another cell some interchanges of nuclear substance took place and the protoplasm was rejuvenated and could again proceed to divide and otherwise show active life.

We may conclude then that simple cell division is an exhausting process, but that the introduction of fresh nuclear substance renews the youth of the protoplasm. Please note that the nucleus and the cell substance may be equally old, but that if they previously belonged to different cells the result is renewed youth.

Some observers have even succeeded in artificially introducing a new nucleus into a broken cell, and the cell has at once shown active powers of growth.

The wear and tear of life then may be partly counteracted by rest or by change of surroundings but a point is at last reached where the only effective means is to dissolve the old relations between a nucleus and its protoplasm, and to interchange them with other cells. The simplest method of doing this is found in those forms of life where a number of cells join together and form a large streaming mass of protoplasm, during which all the nuclei travel up and down in the mass, so that when separation of the cells occurs again they have obtained different nuclei in this game of " general post ".

But when we come to the animals composed of many cells such simple means are impossible. Some cells discharge a purely digestive function, others are nervous, and others are muscular. To play " general post " now would be to reduce the whole body to chaos. The only possibility is to set aside certain cells to which are entrusted this function. These are capable of uniting with a cell of another similar form of life and the result of that union takes on a fresh lease of life and rapidly grows into a new individual.

But we must not imagine that the ordinary cells of the body possess no regenerative capacity. We can, however, definitely state that the cell must possess a nucleus before this is possible. If an Infusorian be cut into several fragments each piece can keep on moving for a time ; but soon the movements slacken and then cease. Each fragment shrinks into a mere spherical drop, except the nucleated one which sets to work and regenerates the whole cell with all its adjuncts again.

One of the labours of Hercules was to slay the many-headed dragon Hydra. As fast as he cut off one head two others sprang up to take its place. Now there is a little creature living in fresh water that rivals the powers of that fabled beast, and therefore it has been given the same name. If it be cut into many pieces, each piece will grow into a new Hydra. It has been even literally turned inside out without doing more than temporarily inconveniencing it ! But the higher we go in the animal kingdom the more limited this power becomes. A star-fish that has accidentally lost an arm can form a new one, a lobster or a crab that has lost a claw, as it frequently does when casting its shell, can replace it, but neither that arm nor that claw can grow into a new star-fish or crab. A lizard can shed its tail piecemeal and grow a new one, but if it loses a leg it cannot grow another. In the higher animals no limb or even part of a limb that has been lost can grow again—we cannot replace even a lost finger or toe. The more complex the animal, the more limited its power of regenerating lost parts, the more nature looks forward to the next generation, and the less she attempts to patch up the old. Therefore it comes about that we have to pay the penalty of our increasing complexity—the different parts of the bodily machine become more closely dependent on each other, and a failure of one part can lead to complete disorganization of the whole.

The chain of life snaps at its weakest link. Were it not so our fate would be that of the famous " one hoss shay " which the logical Deacon made equally strong all over so that nothing could give way first. And the result was that it went to pieces all at once.

Of course a limited local death of certain tissues need not be fatal. The stoppage of the blood supply to any part will cause the death of that part, yet if it contain no vital structures and is not too extensive we may survive it. Thus mortification of a toe from frost-bite or some other cause may lead to loss of that toe but not to loss of life necessarily. Mortification of the whole leg will jeopardize the life but recovery is not impossible. More or less extensive death of bones may occur without fatal results—the body treats the dead bones just as it would a foreign body that had got in by mistake, and makes strenuous attempts to evict it from its place. But without the occurrence of this local death we see a cessation of growth, a tendency to decay, an incapacity for work, following the ageing of the protoplasm which inevitably results from the continued give and take between nucleus and cell substance. It is said, I know not on what authority, that every cell in our body is changed within seven years. I imagine this is well within the mark—probably the life of any cell is of much shorter duration. The duration of the life of the individual will be regulated by the number of times each cell can be replaced when worn out. But this replacement occurs by simple cell division which I have shown to be an exhausting process. It is inevitable that the replacement should begin to be incomplete and unsatisfactory, and it is surprising how soon this downward tendency begins to show itself. " The power of growth diminishes continually though somewhat irregularly throughout life," if we calculate it by the fraction of the total weight which is added to the weight in a given time. At last a point is reached where the curve of growth cuts the base line and the increase becomes a decrease. With the impetus derived at birth we start rolling up the hill of life at an ever lessening pace, for a moment we pause, and then as surely we descend downhill, gathering speed again. But the turning points of the several tissues and organs do not coincide. The gland called the thymus completes its growth in our second year and then begins to shrink. The skeleton is complete in our twenty-fifth year and its very firmness is a portent for the future. For as we shall

297

see the replacement of elastic tissues by rigid ones is one of the characteristics of old age. Growth in stature is no longer possible—in a physical sense it is true that " the prison house begins to close upon the growing boy ". In quite early life, too, the changing of colour or the falling of the hair often brings an autumnal suggestion. And though we may bear this with equanimity, the decline of the eyesight which occurs soon after forty needs more philosophy. For, as Michael Foster said : " The eye is in its prime in childhood when its media are clearest and its mechanisms most mobile, and then it for the most part serves as a toy ; in later years when it could be of the greatest service to a still active brain it has already fallen into a clouded and rigid old age." All this occurs while we feel ourselves to be still in our prime, yet many of the features of old age must depend on this disarrangement of the whole organism produced by the premature decay or disappearance of one or other part. " The future decline of the brain is probably involved in the early decay of the thymus."

To all this we must add the constant attacks to which we are exposed from the outside world—each little trivial scar we bear means some slight defect in the process of repair. As Sir George Humphry used to say, shaking a long forefinger : " Nothing ever gets quite well." And as life goes on the repair gets less and less complete. To quote Foster again : " Everywhere we see a disposition on the part of the living substance of the tissue to fall back on the easier task of forming fat (or calcareous, i.e. chalky material) rather than to carry on the more arduous duty of manufacturing new material like itself." These changes are well seen in the cartilages of the ribs —where the cells become mere fat globules and the supple matrix becomes rigid with chalky deposits ; " the signs of past and the cause of future nutritive decline." This loss of elasticity is, as I have said, most characteristic of old age, and in the blood vessels the result is disastrous. Henceforth the stream of nourishment is no longer conveyed in flexible arteries delicately susceptible to our ever varying needs, but in a rigid tube whose tortuous throbbing on the forehead is a sign that all can read. This change occurs at different ages in different people, which has led to the saying : " A man's as old as his arteries."

The perfection that follows practice, according to Herbert Spencer, is due to the training of nervous currents to run along accustomed channels, instead of wandering into by-paths. But a point is reached when the nervous current can only go along such a channel ; the old work is still done as well, but new work cannot be undertaken. Versatility is lost until the " brain becomes a more or less rigid mass of nervous substance the lines of which rather mark the history of past actions than serve as indications of present potency ".

Thus old men live in the past, for the past ploughed his brain when it was " wax to receive and marble to retain " while the present can make no mark on that marble surface. Even this brings its compensations— the brain no longer worries the stomach but leaves it to discharge its functions undisturbed, and the man who was a " martyr to dyspepsia " in his prime " eats and drinks with the courage and success of a boy ". Fortunately we are but imperfectly conscious of all this, as Sir James Paget found in his masterly analysis of his own old age. " No man over seventy," said he, " walks with the same pliant, elastic, easy step as he walked at thirty or forty, but many over seventy I think are not conscious of the change ; they can see it in others, they cannot feel it in themselves. Anyone I suppose could discern the difference in voice and speech of a friend over seventy while he remembers what it was twenty or thirty years before ; but to the old man himself, I suspect, the change is often imperceptible. He does not observe the diminished range of notes or the veiled sound of his " S " or, worse still, its shrill whistle. It is only when he puts these and the like things to a careful test that he finds the change. He may find it by timing his walk— his full speed may be half a mile less in the hour ; or by trying his voice—he cannot reach his former highest or lowest notes or sustain any note so long as once he could. And so it is throughout ; the change has been so gradual that even the accumulated contrast can be discerned."

Here we have portrayed the sixth age, the " big manly voice turning again towards childish treble, pipes and whistles in his sound ". But the " last stage of all that ends this strange eventful history ", the " mere oblivion " the " sans everything " is rare. The machine is too complex to withstand these repeated insults, the silver cord is loosed, the tripod of life is overturned. This tripod is formed by the heart, the lungs, and the brain. According to Bichat there are three ways of dying—if the heart fails it is syncope, if the lungs asphyxia, and if the brain coma. Yet these are not really independent of one another and the essential feature in all of them is the stoppage of the heart—the circulation comes to an end and the nourishment of all the tissues fails. When the heart stops beyond recovery we say the body is dead ; but we must remember that the individual tissues are not yet dead. The liver can still go on making sugar, the muscles can still respond to stimulation ; according to some the hair can still grow. Just as there may be local death in a living body, so there may be local life in a dead body. At a variable time after the death of the individual the muscles pass into a rigid condition in which they fail to respond to any stimulation, and this has been taken as the sign of their death. And as Foster said: " In all cases it is obvious that the possibility of recovery depending as it does on the skill and knowledge of the experimenter is a wholly artificial sign of death. Yet we can draw no other sharp line between the seemingly dead tissue whose life has flickered down to a mouldering ember which can still be fanned back again into flame and the handful of dust, the aggregate of chemical substances into which the decomposing tissue finally crumbles."

But nature does not stop here. It is usual to speak of

her regal profusion, her reckless prodigality. But though she is lavish she is like a far-seeing investor, not a wasteful spendthrift, she looks to the future. The material is used again, as Omar Khayyam knew.

You may retort that the beauty of the roses is no compensation for the loss of a Cæsar, but the answer is ready at hand—the type is preserved. Millions of seeds are scattered broadcast in order that a few may fall upon good ground. But mark well—some *do* fall upon good ground. What does it matter to Nature so long as she preserves the best types—the raw material can be used over and over again—but she keeps with the utmost care the moulds in which that material is to be re-cast. There is no waste. If we would understand anything of Nature's methods we must turn our eyes from the individual to the race. Let me quote an instance. Look at the elaborate provision insects make for offspring they will never see. " Certain wasps have the habit of stinging the larvæ of beetles in their nerve centres in such a manner as to paralyse their victims without actually killing them. On the body of the paralysed larva a single egg is laid by the wasp and then left to its fate. From the egg a grub is hatched in due time which at once begins to suck the juices of the larva ; the victim supplying it with food sufficient for the whole time of its development. The grub changes into a pupa on the skin of its victim and passing through the winter in the pupa state emerges in the spring as a wasp with the same instincts and habits as its parent. Difficulty is sometimes felt in accounting for such instincts. The individual it is true derives no advantage whatever from its ingenuity ; but the gain to the species is enormous ; and the possession of the habit is due to the fact that those individuals which took the greatest care to make provision for their young would be most likely to give rise to offspring which would survive in the struggle for existence." Nowhere do we see this more clearly than in the marvellously complex civilization of the beehive. From the bee she demands more than provision, she

requires sacrifice. Maeterlinck, in his fascinating book
The Life of the Bee, calls this imperious, unseen Mistress
" The Spirit of the Hive ". And how it dominates all.
" In accordance with the generosity of the season and the
age of the flowers . . . will it permit or forbid the first-
born of the royal princesses to slay in their cradles her
younger sisters, who are singing the song of the Queens.
At other times when the season wanes and the flowery
hours grow shorter it will command the workers themselves to slaughter the whole imperial brood, that the
era of revolutions may close and work becomes the sole
object of all. . . . When the flowers begin to close sooner
and open later the spirit will one morning coldly decree
the simultaneous and general massacre of every male. . . .
Finally it is the spirit of the hive that fixes the hour of
the great annual sacrifice to the genius of the race—the
hour, that is, of the swarm, when we find a whole people
who have attained the topmost pinnacle of prosperity and
power suddenly abandon to the generation to come their
wealth and their palaces their homes and the fruits of
their labour ; themselves content to encounter the hard-
ships and perils of a new and distant country. This act,
be it conscious or not, undoubtedly passes the limits of
human morality. Its result will sometimes be ruin, but
poverty always and the thrice happy city is scattered
abroad in obedience to a law superior to its own happiness.
. . . Where, in what assembly, what intellectual and moral
sphere does this spirit reside to whom all must submit,
itself being vassal to an heroic duty, to an intelligence
whose eyes are persistently fixed on the future." Nature
exacts more from the bees than from man. But from both
she demands the toll of death. Here, too, it has been argued
the solution is to be found in the advantage of the species.
Weismann has brought forward this theory in the
following words: " Let us imagine that one of the higher
animals becomes immortal ; it then becomes perfectly
obvious that it would cease to be of value to the species
to which it belonged. Suppose that such an immortal
individual could escape all fatal accidents through

infinite time—a supposition which is, of course, hardly conceivable. The individual would nevertheless be unable to avoid from time to time slight injuries to one or other parts of its body. The injured parts could not regain their former integrity, and thus the longer the individual lived the more defective and crippled it would become, and the less perfectly would it fulfil the purpose of its species. . . . Worn out individuals are not only valueless to the species but they are even harmful, for they take the place of those which are sound. Hence by the operation of natural selection life would be shortened by the amount which was useless to the species. It would be reduced to a length which would afford the most favourable conditions for the existence of as large a number as possible of vigorous individuals at the same time." Somewhat the same idea had been expressed 150 years before by Dean Swift with all his accustomed power. Gulliver, in his travels, found at Laputa a race among whom immortals were occasionally born. How happy their lot he thought and how enviable. But he found that " the question was not whether a man would choose to be always in the prime of youth attended with prosperity and health ; but how he would pass a perpetual life under all the disadvantages which old age brings along with it. . . . When they came to fourscore years, which is reckoned the extremity of living in this country, they had not only all the follies and infirmities of other old men but many more which arose from the prospect of never dying. . . . They lament and repine that others are gone to a harbour of rest to which they them-selves can never hope to arrive. They have no remem-brance of anything but what they learned and observed in their youth and even that is very imperfect. . . . They were the most mortifying sight I ever beheld . . . and from what I had heard and seen my keen appetite for perpetuity of life was much abated."

Tennyson with his gentler touch, deals with the same subject in his *Legend of Tithonus*, a mortal to whom Jupiter granted eternal life :

" I asked thee ' Give me immortality '
Then did thou grant mine asking with a smile
Like wealthy men who care not how they give
But thy strong Hours indignant worked their will
And beat me down and marred and wasted me
And though they could not end me, left me maimed
. . . And all I was in ashes.

"Take back thy gift
Why should a man desire in any way
To vary from the kindly race of men
Or pass beyond the goal of ordinance
Where all should pause as is most meet for all."

Surely we may feel with Swift—from what we can hear
and see our keen appetite for perpetuity of life may
be much abated. Still the feeling returns, if protoplasm
is immortal why cannot we renew our youth like the
humbler forms of life. Protoplasm can be rejuvenated by
altering the nucleus contained in the cell. But do we
realize what this would entail ? It would mean the
loss of individuality. Though we often envy what another
man has, we never want to *be* that man. We want to
remain ourselves and have his belongings. We cling to
our own individuality. But by the methods of physical
immortality I have described we should be thrown, as
it were, into the melting pot. Our original protoplasm is
seamed and scarred by events and thoughts just as the
coastline is fretted into bays and promontories by the
waves of the sea. Do we wish to lose all that—with our
memories and hopes would go our real selves. What
pleasure then in a fresh unfurrowed brain. Should we
not then cry again with Tithonus—" Take back thy gift."
" The woods decay, the woods decay and die " was his
longing lament. An inexorable limit is set to man's
egoism ; only if blended with another personality can he
go on and renew his youth. The individual who would
live alone shall surely die. Nature has devised a more
excellent way, conserving individuality by handing it on,
as we can clearly see in a gallery of family portraits.

We may say then that death has been evolved for the good of the race, to remove worn out structures in favour of more active ones. And death being thus merely the servant of life, life ultimately attains the mastery over death.

Life can make all things new, and what are our puny interests compared with those of the race? Would we be less far seeing than the bees with " eyes persistently fixed upon the future ".

RETROSPECT

A consulting physician to a hospital has a position of great dignity but of no importance. When I was on the active staff I always tried to be particularly polite to members of the consulting staff on their occasional visits. I thought they were dead without knowing it. Then came the " abhorred shears " and cut me off. Somewhat to my surprise I felt that I was nevertheless still alive ; indeed in some respects more so. I had come to regard the life of the hospital in which more than half my days had been spent as the very hub of existence. Although there was still not much time to " stand and stare " there was more opportunity of gaining wider impressions of life as a whole. It is one of the many compensations of growing older that in middle age one can watch with increasing interest the spacing out of one's contemporaries at school and college in the race of life. Now I could lean over the rails and look at the race from outside, all passion spent as far as competition goes. Moreover it was a pleasing thought that as no one would now be advantaged by my death, no one would presumably wish for it.

I am not troubled by the painful feeling : " If only I had my time over again," and that not because of smug self-satisfaction. Of course I would have preferred to have done many things differently, but should I, given a second chance ? That assumes one could use painfully gained experience to avoid similar mistakes. Barrie showed us otherwise in *Dear Brutus*. But quite apart from this, do I want to repeat the flea-bitten experiences of an extern midwifery clerk ? which by the way gave me a valuable insight into the lives of the very poor. Do I want again to attend to Saturday night " drunks " in the Casualty Department ? The answer is not in doubt. Do I want to undergo again the terrors of examinations ? A distinguished professor told me that he often had nightmares of missing a First in his Tripos for twelve years afterwards. That tells its own tale. Do *you* really want to go back? Some do; Sir Clifford Allbutt, one of my distinguished predecessors in the Regius Chair at Cambridge, wrote to me when nearly ninety years of age :—" I know, rather than feel, that I must be nearing the end of a long life. . . . With all this new knowledge coming up on the horizon what a joy it would be to begin it all over again."

I shall try to avoid discussing the changes I have seen ; we seniors love to do it and when it does not bore our juniors it gives them the impression that we were trained in the dark ages. In the retrospect the span of one's own experience seems astonishingly short ; one can be helped to realize its length by measuring an equal span backwards from the same starting point and seeing what was the state of things then. Taking the date of my birth and sweeping backward thus I find Napoleon I at the height of his power and the battle of Trafalgar yet to be won. I started the study of medicine forty-nine years ago ; an equivalent distance backwards lands us midway between the discoveries of Bright and Addison. Cellular Pathology and the Origin of Species were not due for nearly another twenty years. Another impression derived from this mental exercise is how much more remote things seem which happened before our time than those which happened during our own lifetime.

*   *   *   *   *

Wordsworth " grew old in an age he condemned ", and it has been suggested that we are gently prepared for our exit from this world by the inevitable changes which gradually make us feel less at home in it. I think there is something in this when one finds modern music a choice between discordant cacophony and epileptic negroid croonings, modern sculpture meaningless distortion, modern pictures hideous in colour and design, and modern poetry an unintelligible crossword puzzle. I don't feel at home with stark modern furniture and I don't like its dreary coverings of zigzags in various drab shades of brown. One is still allowed to admire Mozart and Chippendale, however, even if one must only read Tennyson in secret ! When I contrast the magnificent outburst of art in Periclean Athens after the Persian War with the vapourings of modern art since the Great War, I am tempted to speculate on the underlying psychological factors. The Greeks were filled with optimism, the present age is sick with apprehension. This may be largely due to that increased awareness which is the note of the twentieth century. Readers of Jane Austen and her contemporaries have often commented how little their books are tinged with the wars and rumours of wars amid which they were produced. How much is one part of this awareness, that of outside perils, maintained through the hour by hour information poured out by the daily press from all over the world ?

To-day the sword is not being beaten into a ploughshare—rather do hangars arise where once corn grew. Each nation fears another ; many individuals fear shut-in places, while others fear open spaces. Many try to find escape by speed, but what is the good of crossing the Atlantic at a record speed if you are equally unhappy in New York and in London ? No speed will enable us to escape from ourselves.

The effect of all this on the younger generation is sometimes quite serious. C. P. Snow in his novel, *The Search*, describes this effect upon the lives of a group of research workers. He makes one of them say, " Your father and mother hadn't the certainty more or less that civilization is going to crash in their lifetime. We have. . . . For you and me, for almost everyone life is fuller and richer than it has ever been. With one qualification. There is no hope. . . . Simple freedoms, but very precious . . . my sort of man has only had for an infinitesimally short time. They'll have gone from all over Europe except France and England and Scandinavia in ten years. From England in twenty. And for a very long time they will not come again."

We may think this picture is too black ; the important

thing is that it represents a not uncommon point of view and it is one which must tend to paralyse endeavour.

"Age and crabbèd youth cannot live together." Thus H. W. Nevinson inverted Shakespeare's line, after reading "The Voice of Under Thirty" in the *Spectator* lately. Many readers were distressed at the indecision and despair most of these youthful writers betrayed. But this is really nothing new. I remember that before the War the sea-green, incorruptible *Westminster Gazette* published a series of articles entitled "Si jeunesse savait", much to the same effect. I have cheered many a gloomy adolescent by referring him to the preface of Keats' *Endymion*, wherein he says that between boyhood and maturity "there is a space of life in which the soul is in a ferment, the character undecided, the way of life uncertain, the ambition thick-sighted ; thence proceeds mawkishness and . . . [a] thousand bitters". It is reassuring for such a one to find that Keats, who accomplished so much, felt as he does now.

No doubt such feelings often find expression in a form which we seniors find distinctly unpleasing, but if we look back at our own youth we must in candour admit that our seniors must often have found us disagreeable while we were trying to assert our individuality. And we must remember that we grew up in a world which seemed relatively sane and stable.

*   *   *   *   *

Robert Louis Stevenson said that it happened he had the very last of the very best of his old University which was the more strange as the same thing befell his father before him, and if he had a son, doubtless it would also be his fate. This frame of mind exists because being at the University is like falling in love ; no one can ever have had such an experience before, nor is it credible that anyone else can have it in the future.

My love for my own University, unlike so many early loves, has never faltered, but rather grown with the years. "Sir," said Dr. Johnson, "the finest prospect to a

Scotsman is the road which leads to England." To me the finest prospect is the road that is sign-posted to Cambridge. Or coming by rail, the authentic thrill begins when the train draws up at the long, unlovely platform. What is it about one's University that colours the whole of the rest of life? True one discovers oneself, but can the discovery of a very ordinary individual by himself have this magic effect? Is it not rather the discovery of oneself in relation to the general scheme of things, the realization of being a small part of something greater, which was there before us and will outlast us? It may be urged that this is the lesson of the public school. Perhaps; but the number of things in which it is correct to be interested at school is severely restricted by the pressure of the herd. The first impression at the University is the sensation of release from taboos. It has its own taboos of course, but they are not nearly so limiting in their effect. I went to Cambridge shy, awkward, and diffident, though extremely ambitious; I met with the most kindly encouragement—what germs of promise my teachers cunningly detected, they assiduously cultivated. But that is by no means all; my friend Professor Ernest Barker recently said, " Ideals must become flesh and dwell in persons in order to be freely followed. Mind must be put to mind in free intercourse in order to maintain a real unity of minds." And as that loyal son of Cambridge, Augustine Birrell, wrote, " It is within the crumbling walls of old colleges that mind meets with mind, that permanent friendships are formed, habits of early rising contracted, lofty ambitions stirred. It is indeed a great and a stirring tradition. Who does not recall the neat little banquets in the monastic cells? Which of us who is clad in the sober russet of middle life can gaze without emotion upon the old break-neck staircase in the corner of an ancient quadrangle where once he kept, and where were housed for a too brief season the bright-coloured, long-since abandoned garments of a youth apparently endless, and of hopes that knew no bounds? " Another Cambridge

man, Lowes Dickinson, beautifully expressed that sense
of continuity and perpetual youth thus :—" Others of
that set have gone almost out of my mind, and some of
them out of the world. But still their forms appear in
the golden mists of dawn and almost I catch their voices
through talk of younger generations, heard under the
same chapel walls and the same chestnut groves, on the
same great lawns, under the same stars, reflected in
the same sluggish yet lovely stream that will hear perhaps
for centuries yet the same voices at the same budding time
of youth." That is what R. L. S. meant by each of us
having the very last of the very best, for it is our own for
the rest of our lives.

At a rational level, however, one knows that in many
ways things have improved at the Universities, though
one doubts if the student can now lead so care-free an
existence. But one great difference I do notice. In my
time every college was honeycombed with little discussion
societies, where aided by coffee and " whales on toast "
we criticized a paper read by one of our number. To-day
few such societies seem to exist—" if we have some time
off, we go to the cinema " one undergraduate told me—
and such societies as do exist prefer to get a senior man
to read the paper. Student medical societies too often
do the same. What a valuable training they are missing.
I always look back with pleasure to those " Noctes
Ambrosianæ " when having

" tired the Sun with talking and sent him down the sky "

we put the world to rights. This education of one
another by ourselves was surely one of the most valuable
things in University life. Yet a young Oxford novelist,
David Winser, makes a character say, " With no one have
I sat in front of the fire and talked into the small hours.
And my uncles used to. Almost every night. No one at
all except a Groupist. And even then it wasn't me who
was talking." I can hardly credit it, however, that
undergraduates have ceased to talk !

*   *   *   *   *

Amid the disquiet and clamour of the day I turn with relief to the advance of medicine. Despite some disagreeable eddies and unsavoury backwaters, its main stream runs clear and sweeps onward with a gathering impetus. It is, I think, helpful to look at life in general from the special angle provided by a medical training; helpful also to the community, if thereby some of the symptoms of the " general malaise" so prevalent to-day can be interpreted. How interesting it would be to have a modern version of Sir Thomas Browne's *Enquiries into Vulgar and Common Errors*. For though we should be less inclined than he to regard Satan as the invisible agent and secret promoter who plays in the dark without us, we should cordially agree that the seed of error is within ourselves.

What, for instance, is the origin of the popular belief in the safety and harmlessness of " herbal remedies " in spite of the fact that some of the deadliest poisons are of vegetable origin ? The very name " deadly nightshade " is not reassuring ; the savage poisons his arrow tips with " the hellish ourali ", and a cup of hemlock silenced the wisdom of Socrates. Yet I read in a herbalist pamphlet that " the Herbs provided by benevolent Nature " help to maintain a high standard of physical health because they are grown in the fresh air and sunshine and are therefore full of vital properties. Which should be a consoling reflection to a man in the convulsive torments of strychnine poisoning. If " benevolent Nature " placed the helpful alkaloids in plants, who put the poisonous ones there ? Next we are informed that the machine age cut us off from our age-old Nature medicines. This does something less than justice to the chemists and pharmacologists who isolated the active principles from these herbs in a pure form, separated the good from the evil, and substituted precise dosage for infusions and tisanes of vague and variable strength. I fail to see why vegetable drugs are the most " natural " for animals. Surely the most natural drugs for them are those produced by their own bodies, the hormones and anti-toxins. Why such products should be called filthy and herbal remedies natural is even more unintelligible to me than Bunthorne's alleged passion for " a vegetable love ".

I distrust all quasi-medical slogans, whether, " Herbs are Nature's remedy," " like cures like," " pain is a false claim " or " the osteopathic lesion ". Incidentally they are mutually exclusive. To me they indicate a pathetic craving for certainty in this uncertain world. It is not without significance that such cults have increased just when science has become less dogmatic. I have been comparing Carl Snyder's *New Conceptions in Science*, published in 1903, with J. W. Sullivan's *Limitations of Science*, published in 1933. The cocksure materialism of the earlier work is completely lacking in the later one. It is curious that with the evaporation of this from scientific thought there should be in the world of affairs such a renewed belief in the fallacy of force. Violence is preferred to reason. In the early days of this century, woman, who is traditionally accredited with superior intuition, sensed this change was coming and realized that the suffrage which had been denied to reason would be granted to violence. Professor Houston has given an interesting medical illustration of the " need for violent action when in distress ". He says " the pride of personality is so strong that many patients would prefer to submit to a dozen surgical operations rather than concede that their troubles are due to a deformity of personality ". Every medical man knows how difficult it is for patients to accept the idea that their ill-health is due to a conflict between their own ego and the environment. Somehow or other, belief in a slogan which proclaims a panacea pleases and comforts the disgruntled ego.

It has been truly said of a distinguished physician who recently passed away that " beneath his interest in the foibles and weakness of his fellows there lay, not a feeling of superiority or scorn, but a kindly pitying tolerance and a great humour ". Indeed if our profession does not teach us tolerance and humour we have practised it in vain. The recognition of the close correlation between the psychological and physical aspects of disease has, I think, encouraged an earlier development of insight into the mental distresses which produce physical symptoms. But indeed we can see evidence of the advance of medicine in every direction, an advance which is so rapid as to leave some of us seniors rather breathless in the attempt to keep pace with it. I am cheered, however, by the reflection that if it was the youthful Samuel who had the vision, the old man Eli was needed to interpret it. I once heard Bishop Paget say of his father's attitude towards Listerian antisepsis that like Moses on Mount Pisgah he saw the Promised Land but knew that he could not enter therein. That was finely said ; it is sometimes well to realise as life goes on, that we must leave things to younger men to accomplish. We may see a new truth, but be too set in our ways to ensue it. It is well to be able to say, " The life to which I belong uses me, and will pass beyond me, and I am content."

INDEX OF NAMES

INDEX OF SUBJECTS

331